LUNG DISORDERS

Peter B. Terry, M.D.

JOHNS HOPKINS
MEDICINE

Dear Readers:

Over this past year, lung disorders have certainly found their way into the headlines. Johnny Carson passed away from emphysema. Peter Jennings died of lung cancer. Dana Reeve was diagnosed with lung cancer despite having never smoked.

But the news hasn't been all bad. This year's Lung Disorders White Paper reports on the most exciting advances and the most useful, current information to help you prevent or treat respiratory diseases. The main text provides a thorough overview of what the medical field knows about lung disorders—their causes, symptoms, diagnostic procedures, and treatment options. The research columns (located in the margins) report on the latest studies—sometimes confirming what we already know, and sometimes questioning our practices and current understanding (as the scientific process so often does). Finally, the dozen or so features (articles located in shaded boxes throughout the White Paper) focus on special topics that we felt warranted particular attention this year.

Here are some of the feature highlights for 2006:

- **Traveling with oxygen**—tips for each mode of transportation. (page 28)
- Tips for **COPD** patients on conserving energy during routine tasks. (page 22)
- When **aggressive treatment** is advisable for elderly **lung cancer** patients. (page 47)
- Treating **sleep apnea** to protect your **heart.** (page 33)
- New research on the effectiveness of **antibiotics** in treating **bronchitis.** (page 55)
- **Medications** that could be making your **asthma** worse. (page 11)
- New research on the dangers of **second-hand smoke**. (page 27)
- **Asthma** increases the risk of **gastroesophageal reflux disease** (GERD). (page 13)
- **Ordering drugs from Canada** to save money? Make sure you're being safe. (page 34)

I hope the information provided in this White Paper will empower you to make informed decisions about your respiratory health.

Sincerely,

Peter B. Terry, M.D.
Professor of Medicine
Division of Pulmonary and Critical Care Medicine
Johns Hopkins University School of Medicine

P. S. Please visit www.HopkinsLung.com for the latest news on lung disorders and other information that will complement your Johns Hopkins White Paper.

THE AUTHOR

Peter B. Terry, M.D., M.A., is a professor of medicine in the Division of Pulmonary and Critical Care Medicine at the Johns Hopkins University School of Medicine. He is also an associate professor in the Department of Anesthesiology/Critical Care Medicine at Johns Hopkins Hospital and an associate professor in the Department of Environmental Health Sciences at the Johns Hopkins School of Public Health. In addition, he is a member of the Berman Bioethics Institute at Johns Hopkins.

Dr. Terry received his M.D. from St. Louis University and subsequently trained at the University of Connecticut, Johns Hopkins Hospital, and the Mayo Clinic. He has a master's degree in philosophy with a concentration in bioethics from The Kennedy Institute of Ethics at Georgetown University.

CONTENTS

LUNG DISORDERS

Disorders of breathing (respiration) are common in the United States and will no doubt become more prevalent as the population ages. More than 300,000 Americans die of lung disease every year, and over 35 million are now living with chronic lung disease. Fortunately, technological advances are producing unprecedented opportunities to prevent, diagnose, and treat respiratory diseases. This has resulted in considerable improvements in the lifespan and quality of life of people suffering from these disorders.

This White Paper provides the latest information on the prevention and treatment of a number of common lung diseases. Our goal is to help you work more closely and effectively with your healthcare providers to improve your breathing. The following disorders are reviewed:

Asthma. Asthma is an inflammatory lung disease characterized by shortness of breath, wheezing, coughing, and tightness in the chest. It is considered an obstructive lung disease because it causes narrowing of the airways. With careful management, most people with asthma can breathe normally and lead otherwise healthy and active lives.

Chronic obstructive pulmonary disease. Chronic obstructive pulmonary disease (COPD) includes chronic bronchitis and emphysema. Like asthma, COPD is an obstructive lung disease. However, the obstruction in COPD is more difficult to manage because of permanent damage to the lungs. Fortunately, there are many steps people with COPD can take to make life easier.

Sleep apnea. Sleep apnea refers to temporary, recurrent breathing interruptions during sleep. Marked daytime drowsiness and snoring are 2 common signs of sleep apnea. People with this disorder can improve both their breathing and their sleeping with the help of today's available treatments.

Interstitial lung disease. Interstitial lung disease refers to a group of conditions that cause extensive scarring of the tissue between the air sacs in the lungs. This tissue is called the interstitium. Although treatment is not always effective, supportive medical care can help people with this condition live more comfortably.

Lung cancer. Lung cancer, which is most often caused by cigarette smoking, is the leading cause of cancer death in the United States. While lung cancer often is not caught before it has spread and becomes difficult to treat, many new therapies are being tested.

How Your Lungs Work: The ABC's of Breathing

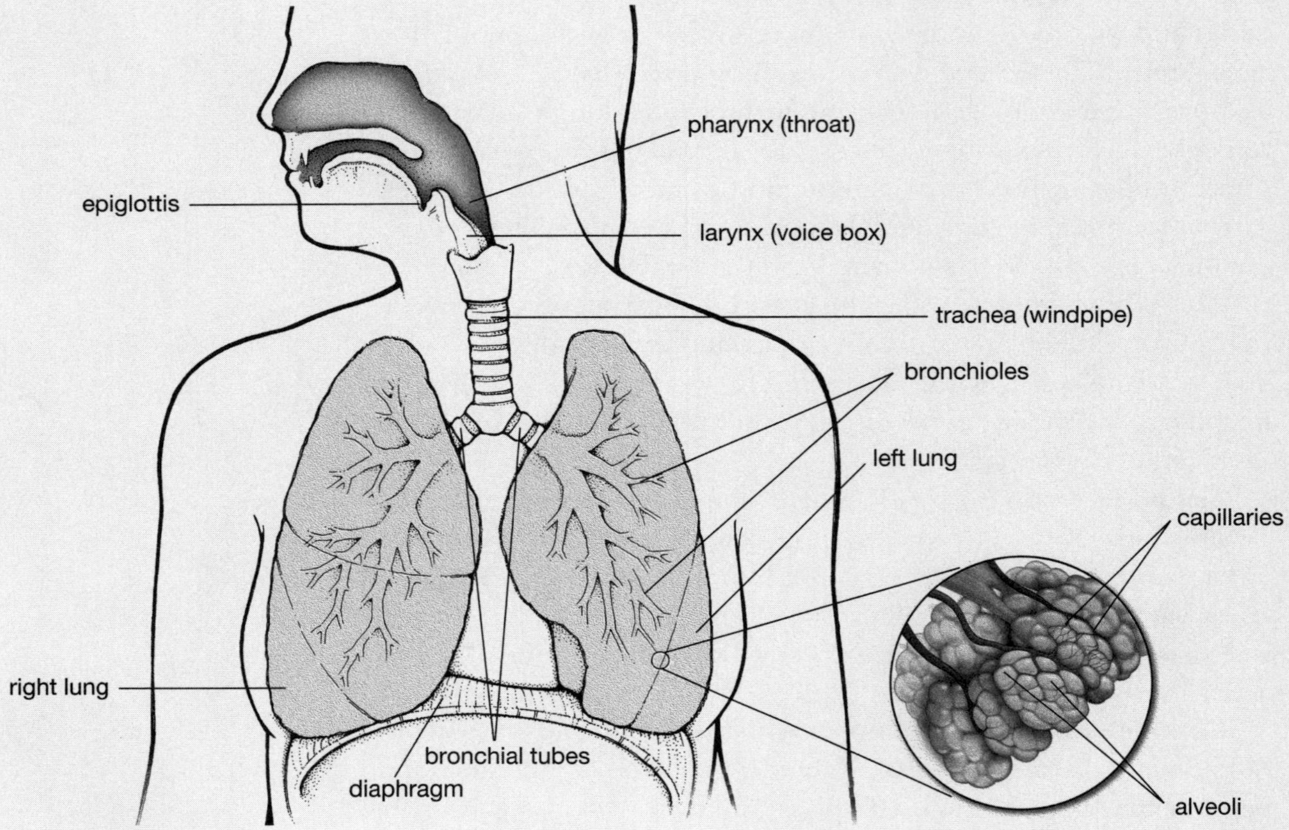

Your lungs make oxygen available to your body and remove other gases, such as carbon dioxide. When you inhale through your nose or mouth, air travels down the back of your throat (pharynx), passes through your voice box (larynx), and into your windpipe (trachea). The trachea is divided into 2 air passages (bronchial tubes); one leads to the left lung, and one to the right lung. The diaphragm, a dome-shaped muscle, lies below the lungs. It flattens to draw air in as you inhale, and rises when you exhale.

The right lung has 3 sections, called lobes, and is slightly larger than the left lung, which has 2 lobes. The bronchial tubes divide into smaller air passages (bronchi), and then into even smaller passages called bronchioles. At the end of the bronchioles are tiny air sacs called alveoli, where oxygen and carbon dioxide are exchanged.

After absorbing oxygen, the blood flows from the lungs to the heart. It is then pumped through the body, providing oxygen to the cells of the tissues and organs. When the cells use the oxygen, carbon dioxide (CO_2) is produced and transferred to the blood. The blood carries the CO_2 back to the lungs, where it is removed when you exhale.

Your lungs are protected from harmful substances in several ways. The hair (cilia) in the nose helps filter out large particles, and cilia in the air passages continually sweep back and forth to keep the air passages clear

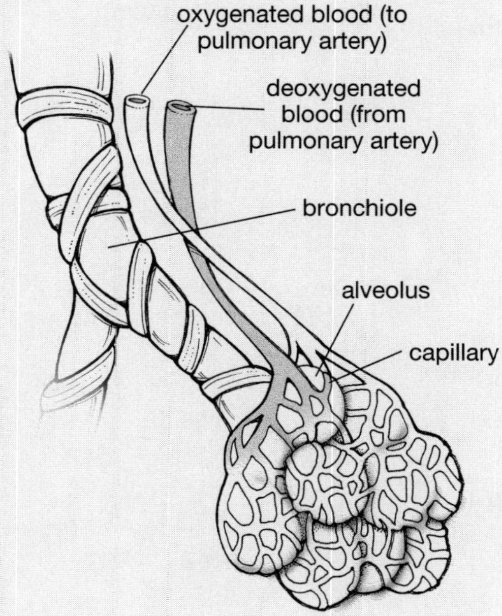

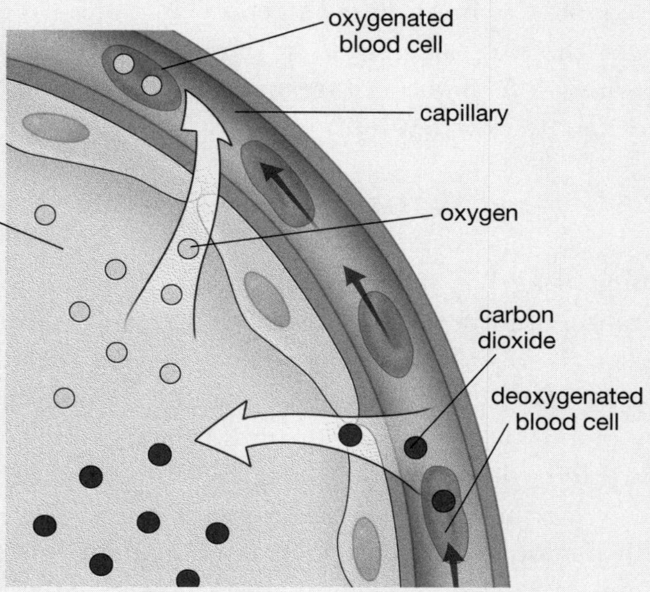

Oxygen and Carbon Dioxide Exchange

(cigarette smoke can damage cilia). Mucus produced by the trachea and bronchial tubes helps trap dust, bacteria, and other foreign substances before they enter the lungs.

In a person with normal breathing, the airways are open and free from inflammation and excess mucus. In asthma, breathing in triggers the lining of the airways to become inflamed and swollen. The lining can make extra mucus, which clogs the airways. The muscles around the airways tighten, making the airways even narrower. Sometimes the airways can become so narrow that air has trouble getting in and out of the lungs, resulting in an asthma attack.

In chronic bronchitis, the lining of the bronchioles becomes inflamed and produces too much mucus. The swelling and excess mucus narrow the airways and restrict airflow in and out of the lungs, causing shortness of breath. The cilia are also damaged, preventing them from removing the excess mucus.

In emphysema, the alveoli are destroyed, making it difficult for the lungs to absorb enough oxygen or rid themselves of enough CO_2. The walls of the alveoli lose their elasticity and become enlarged. As they get bigger, the diaphragm flattens, making it harder for the lungs to move air in and out. The bronchioles also become less elastic, and become narrow or collapse upon exhalation. As a result, CO_2 gets trapped in the airways and prevents oxygen from getting to the blood. ■

Pulmonary embolism. A pulmonary embolism usually occurs when a blood clot from a deep vein in the leg breaks loose and blocks 1 or more arteries within the lungs. A number of treatments are available to prevent blood clots from forming and emboli from becoming life threatening.

Infections. Common lung infections include acute bronchitis, influenza (the flu), and bacterial pneumonia. Vaccines can help prevent these infections, and treatments are available to ease their impact when they do develop.

SYMPTOMS OF RESPIRATORY DISORDERS

Many lung disorders produce similar symptoms, but the severity and duration of these symptoms can vary considerably from disease to disease. The disorders can be acute (short and relatively severe) or chronic (persisting over a long time). Pneumonia and pulmonary embolism are acute lung disorders; asthma, COPD, and interstitial lung disease are chronic disorders. Chronic lung conditions may wax and wane in severity and can worsen quickly and markedly if another problem, such as a lung infection, occurs.

Common symptoms of lung disorders include shortness of breath, coughing, noisy breathing, and chest pain. Some people, however, have only mild symptoms or none at all. In these individuals, the disorder may be detected on a chest x-ray or by a test to check lung function.

Shortness of breath. Shortness of breath can dramatically compromise quality of life. The underlying cause of shortness of breath is usually a mechanical problem in the lungs or diaphragm (the large, dome-shaped muscle located at the base of the lungs). Examples of mechanical problems are airway obstruction (as occurs in asthma, COPD, and some lung cancers); increased stiffness of the lungs (as in interstitial lung disease, pneumonia, and heart failure); severe spine and rib cage abnormalities; and obesity. If left untreated, shortness of breath can lead to fatigue and weakness that may profoundly limit activities. In turn, weakness related to being out of shape or musculoskeletal disease, such as severe curvature of the spine, may aggravate shortness of breath.

Coughing. Coughing up phlegm, infectious germs, and foreign substances is one of the ways in which the lungs protect themselves. Severe coughing, however, may signal a respiratory disease. Obstructive diseases of the lungs (asthma and COPD) and lung cancer often cause a person to cough up phlegm, which, if yellow

NEW RESEARCH

Overweight Women at Higher Risk of Asthma and Allergy

Overweight women have an increased risk of asthma and allergy, but there is no such association in men, according to a new study.

Several studies have found a link between asthma and obesity in women, but it has been unclear whether this association is due to asthma itself or to symptoms caused by being overweight. It is also not known at what age this association develops, or whether it is confined to females.

The researchers studied 1,000 males and females ages 9–26. The body mass index of each participant was measured, and information on asthma, lung function, and allergy was obtained on multiple occasions.

In addition to finding that females—but not males—were at increased risk of asthma and allergy if they were overweight, the researchers found that asthma was not associated with a raised body mass index in childhood, and childhood asthma did not lead to being overweight as an adult.

In summary, a high body mass index is associated with asthma and allergy in women but not men. Moreover, the researchers estimate that 28% of asthma developing in women after age 9 is due to being overweight.

AMERICAN JOURNAL OF RESPIRATORY AND CRITICAL CARE MEDICINE
Volume 171, page 440
March 2005

or green, may signal an infection. Coughing up blood is a critical sign, especially in a current or former cigarette smoker. It may suggest a potentially life-threatening disease, such as lung cancer or pulmonary embolism, although it can also be a sign of a less serious problem such as bronchitis.

Chronic cough in an adult with a normal chest x-ray is most often the result of postnasal drip, asthma, or gastroesophageal reflux (GERD, in which stomach acid flows back into the esophagus; see "Asthma and Reflux" on page 13). Interstitial lung disease, bronchiectasis (persistent widening of the airways), and pneumonia, all of which produce inflammation or scarring of the lungs, also cause coughing.

Noisy breathing. Noisy breathing is an especially common sign of respiratory disease. Abnormal sounds range from a high-pitched crowing during inhalation (which occurs with croup, inflammation of the epiglottis [see illustration on page 2], or tumors in the upper airway) to continuous musical sounds during exhalation (wheezing, which occurs with asthma and some other disorders). The maxim "all that wheezes is not asthma" underscores the fact that many health conditions, including diseases of the larynx, heart failure, pulmonary embolism, and COPD, can cause wheezing. Repetitive loud snoring during sleep, interrupted by periods of silence in which there is no airflow, is a major sign of sleep apnea.

Chest pain. Chest pain or other discomfort has numerous causes, and determining whether the cause is a heart, esophageal, or respiratory disease is often challenging. Pain on one side of the chest that worsens with deep breathing, coughing, or laughing suggests pleurisy, an inflammation of the pleura (the membrane around the surface of the lungs and the inner chest wall). Pleurisy may be caused by a viral infection, pneumonia on the outer surface of the lung, pulmonary embolism, cancer, or a systemic (affecting the entire body) inflammatory disease such as systemic lupus erythematosus. Alternatively, pain that worsens on inhalation may be due to a chest wall injury such as a broken rib.

Other symptoms. Respiratory illnesses also can produce general symptoms. For example, low levels of oxygen in the blood, fragmented sleep patterns, chronic lung infections, and lung cancer can all lead to fatigue. Many people whose respiratory illness limits their daily activities have particular difficulty with activities that involve the arms, such as carrying objects, showering, and performing other grooming tasks. These tasks often become a greater challenge than walking.

NEW RESEARCH

Can Nasal Filters Reduce Hay Fever Symptoms?

Results from the first clinical trial to measure the effectiveness of nasal filters in reducing hay fever symptoms suggest that the devices can significantly improve symptoms.

Researchers studied 46 people with a history of Fall allergies to ragweed or grass pollen. Half the participants were given active nasal filters—soft plastic filter tubes that sit inside the nasal cavities—while the other half were given filters that looked like the nasal filters but lacked an inner core to catch pollen. All study participants spent 2 hours on a Fall day in a park where ragweed and grass pollen counts were high. Symptoms were recorded every 30 minutes.

Participants wearing the active nasal filters had significantly reduced symptoms, including sneezing, runny and itchy nose, sniffles, itchy throat, and itchy and watery eyes, compared with participants wearing the dummy filters. The most noticeable results were seen immediately after participants had spent 20 minutes sitting beside a large patch of ragweed.

Nasal filters may be useful for exposure to perennial allergens, especially those from house dust mites. However, additional studies are needed to examine the feasibility of using the filters for longer periods of time.

ALLERGY
Volume 60, page 529
April 2005

EVALUATION OF RESPIRATORY SYMPTOMS

The first steps in the evaluation of respiratory problems involve a review of your medical history and a physical examination. These will help your doctor, who may be a pulmonologist (a lung specialist), determine which laboratory tests and chest-imaging techniques are needed.

Medical History

Your doctor will ask a number of questions about current symptoms, past behaviors, occupation, toxic exposures (for example, to cigarette smoke, silica [fine dust from quartz], or asbestos), and family medical history. The doctor will also take into account the presence of infections, such as the flu, in the family or community.

Your doctor will want to know if you have ever smoked cigarettes and whether you may have inhaled any other potentially injurious agents, such as asbestos. You will need to give information about any previously diagnosed respiratory illnesses in yourself and your family. You will also discuss any allergies you may have and any medications you take. Sometimes diet pills, amiodarone (Cordarone, used to treat an irregular heart rhythm), or other medications can contribute to lung disease.

In some people, problems that seem unrelated to the lungs—such as skin rash, joint pain, and visual changes—are symptoms of a more generalized inflammatory disease, with respiratory difficulty as one of its symptoms. In addition, a disease such as lung cancer can cause symptoms elsewhere in the body if it spreads.

Physical Examination

The physical examination for a possible lung disease includes a check of breathing rate and pattern and an assessment of how the torso moves during breathing. The way the torso moves is important because some people with lung disease use extra muscles in their abdomen, neck, and rib cage to aid in breathing. Also, reduced movement in one side of the chest might suggest disease in the lung on that side. Finally, abnormalities in the structure of the chest could be the cause of breathing difficulty.

In addition, your doctor will use his or her senses of touch and hearing to evaluate the condition. Touching the chest wall may reveal rib fractures or other sources of chest pain. Percussion (tapping to generate sound) of the chest will help your doctor determine how far the diaphragm moves and how much the lungs

A Dictionary of Doctors Involved in Lung Care

> "My patients often ask why they are seeing so many doctors. A person with lung cancer, for example, may start with their internist, be referred to a pulmonologist, then to an oncologist, thoracic surgeon, radiologist, and pathologist. These specialists all have important and distinct roles in the individual's care."
>
> —**Peter B. Terry, M.D., M.A.**
> (author of this White Paper)

If you have a serious lung disorder, you may see several specialists during the course of your treatment. You may suddenly find yourself dealing with 2 or more specialists at once and have questions about which doctor does what. This happens even to patients who are medically savvy. The following is a quick guide to specialists whom you may encounter.

Internist
A medical doctor who specializes in the care of adults. Internists often serve as primary care doctors, performing regular checkups and treating routine illnesses. If you have a lung disorder, your internist may refer you to a specialist such as a pulmonologist or allergist/immunologist for specialized care.

Pulmonologist
These are specialists who are trained in diseases and conditions of the lungs and airways, such as pneumonia, asthma, emphysema, tuberculosis, or complicated chest infections. Pulmonologists do not perform surgery, but do perform specialized procedures to obtain samples of the lining of the chest wall or the lung. For example, during a bronchoscopy, pulmonologists use flexible fiber optics to see inside the air passages and extract samples for study. They also perform angiographic visualization—injecting dye into the pulmonary arteries to view the blood vessels in the lungs.

Allergist/Immunologist
These types of doctors specialize in the prevention, diagnosis, and treatment of disorders of the human immune system. Such conditions include asthma; rhinitis (inflammation in the lining of the nose); eczema (skin inflammation); and adverse reactions to drugs, foods, and insect stings. They also deal with immune deficiency diseases (both acquired and at birth), defects in the immune system, malignancies of the immune system, and organ transplantation issues.

When it comes to asthma, an allergist can use a series of tests to identify some of an individual's specific triggers. Knowing what triggers your asthma is a critical step in managing it.

Medical Oncologist
Oncologists specialize in the diagnosis and treatment of all types of cancers and tumors. They can order and administer chemotherapy for treating malignant cancers and consult with surgeons and radiologists on other cancer treatments.

Thoracic Surgeon
These doctors provide surgical care of the lungs, coronary arteries, esophagus, and chest wall. They can treat abnormalities of the trachea, the great vessels, and the heart valves, as well as diseases of the diaphragm.

Radiologist
These specialists use techniques such as x-rays, ultrasound, magnetic resonance imaging (MRI), computerized tomography (CT) scan, nuclear medicine, and image-guided interventional procedures to visualize the body and its organs, aiding in the diagnosis and treatment of diseases.

Pathologist
Pathology is a medical specialty focused on making a definitive diagnosis of various diseases, including cancer. Pathologists identify diseases by studying cells and tissues under a microscope and writing a report detailing the diagnosis, which helps the treating physician decide on a course of action. The referring physician usually deals directly with the pathologist (the patient seldom meets the pathologist). ■

inflate during breathing. Your doctor will also listen to breath sounds using a stethoscope.

Examination of the hands may reveal discoloration of the nail beds or clubbing of the fingers (a thickening of the fingertips and increased curvature of the fingernails). Blue nail beds suggest low levels of oxygen in the blood, while clubbing suggests lung cancer, interstitial lung disease, bronchiectasis (persistent widening of the airways), or other problems. Swelling of the legs and feet suggests that a heart problem may be the cause of symptoms. Heart failure can cause difficulty breathing, as can a heart condition known as cor pulmonale, which is caused by high blood pressure in the lungs. Swelling in one leg suggests a blood clot, which could potentially lead to pulmonary embolism (a blockage in the lung).

Medical Tests

Your doctor may order a blood test to look for clues such as anemia (a low red blood cell count), which might explain shortness of breath or suggest a chronic condition such as lung cancer. A blood test might also reveal an elevated white blood cell count, which might suggest a lung infection.

In addition to blood tests, chest imaging and pulmonary function tests are 2 other diagnostic tools that are commonly used to evaluate people suspected of having a lung disorder. Chest imaging provides information primarily about the structure of the lungs and chest, while pulmonary function tests measure lung function. The 2 tests complement each other.

Chest imaging. A chest x-ray may reveal an abnormality that may clearly explain the respiratory problem or may flag areas for further evaluation. Lung tumors, pneumonia, occupational lung diseases, emphysema, interstitial lung disease, and collection of fluid in the lungs can all be seen on a chest x-ray. A chest computed tomography (CT) scan provides a more detailed assessment of abnormalities than a standard chest x-ray. In addition, combination positron emission tomography (PET) and CT scans are now being used to determine the presence of lung cancer. Comparing current chest images with previous images is extremely important, as this can help distinguish a new disease from a pre-existing condition as well as monitor the progression of a disease over time.

Pulmonary function tests. Pulmonary function tests measure lung capacity and reveal patterns characteristic of particular diseases. A person's measurements are compared with those expected for a healthy person of the same age, height, and gender. The tests can help characterize the lung abnormality as primarily obstructive (in which the airways are narrowed), primarily restrictive (in which the ability of the lungs to expand is impaired), or a combination of the 2. The tests also determine whether the deficit in lung function is mild, moderate, or severe.

Commonly performed pulmonary function tests include spirometry, lung volume tests, and diffusion capacity tests. Spirometry, in which a person breathes into a tube attached to a machine called a spirometer, measures the volume of air that can be exhaled and the rate of exhalation. The 2 most important values are the forced expiratory volume in 1 second (FEV_1) and the forced vital capacity (FVC). FEV_1 measures the amount of air expelled from the lungs in the first second of a forced exhalation, while FVC is a measure of the total volume of air exhaled. These values are calculated automatically by the spirometer, along with the ratio comparing the amount of air exhaled in the first second with the total amount of air exhaled: FEV_1/FVC.

Exercise testing. Exercise testing using a treadmill or stationary bicycle may be used to evaluate shortness of breath and to determine whether it is caused by a lung problem, heart disease, or simply being out of shape.

Blood gases. If the lungs are not functioning properly, the amount of oxygen and carbon dioxide in the blood (blood gases) may be affected. Blood gases can be measured by taking a sample of blood from an artery. Alternatively, pulse oximetry provides a noninvasive way to measure the level of oxygen in the blood. In pulse oximetry, a sensor that directs a beam of light through the tissue is placed on the fingertip or earlobe. The sensor monitors oxygen levels in the blood by measuring the amount of light absorbed by the oxygen-carrying pigment in red blood cells (hemoglobin).

APPROACHES TO DISEASE MANAGEMENT

Usually, the general evaluation just described provides enough information to diagnose a lung disorder and devise a management plan. Sometimes, however, the initial evaluation does not provide a definitive diagnosis. If this is the case, invasive procedures to obtain biopsy samples of cells and tissues may be necessary. For example, when fluid collects in the space around the lung, it may be extracted with a needle and analyzed in a lab. Removal of the fluid may help relieve shortness of breath.

Treating someone with a respiratory illness, as with any illness, involves weighing the risks and benefits of each treatment option and taking the patient's personal preferences into account. A cure is available for many lung disorders, including many caused by infections. For all lung disorders, treatment is available to help relieve symptoms.

NEW RESEARCH

Depression Common in People with Chronic Cough

More than half of people suffering with chronic cough, which can last for months or even years, also suffer from depressive symptoms, a new study finds.

Researchers evaluated 100 people with chronic cough that had lasted an average of 9 years. They found that 53% suffered from depressive symptoms, with similar rates in men and women.

Three months after the initial study, researchers conducted a follow-up with two-thirds of the original participants. They found that those whose cough improved had a significant reduction in depressive symptoms, while those whose cough did not get better showed no improvements in their depressive symptoms.

Cough is the single most common complaint for which people visit the doctor in the U.S., and this study is the first to examine the link between cough and depression.

Chronic cough has 3 main causes, either alone or in combination—post-nasal drip, asthma, and gastroesophageal reflux (GERD), commonly known as acid reflux. Treatments include older antihistamines combined with decongestants for cough from post-nasal drip; asthma medicines for asthmatic cough; and high doses of drugs called proton-pump inhibitors for several months, sometimes combined with other drugs, for GERD-related cough.

AMERICAN THORACIC SOCIETY INTERNATIONAL CONFERENCE
Abstract 255
May 2005

OBSTRUCTIVE DISEASES OF THE LUNGS

Asthma and chronic obstructive pulmonary disease (COPD) are obstructive lung diseases, meaning they are characterized by a narrowing of the airways that obstructs airflow when a person exhales. In asthma, the obstruction tends to be intermittent and reversible, but in COPD, it is unremitting and less responsive to medication.

Asthma

Asthma is a chronic inflammatory disorder of the airways. It is the eighth most common chronic condition in the United States, affecting an estimated 20 million Americans. Without proper management and prompt treatment of attacks, asthma can be life threatening. In 2002, more than 4,000 people—mostly seniors—died of the disorder. It has become an increasingly recognized problem in people over the age of 65, who account for about 10% of all people with asthma. Older people tend to have other health problems and more frequent asthmatic symptoms, making appropriate treatment particularly important in this age group.

Causes. Asthma is caused by an immune system abnormality that appears to have genetic and environmental components. The 2 defining features of asthma are inflammation and over-sensitivity (hyper-reactivity) of the airways, both of which lead to obstruction of airflow. Airway inflammation involves swelling of the airway lining and excessive production and accumulation of mucus. These problems can be aggravated by a respiratory infection such as sinusitis, flu, or a cold. Hyper-reactive airways tend to "twitch" when exposed to allergens and other irritants, causing the muscles around the airways to contract involuntarily. Both inflammation and hyper-reactivity cause narrowing of the airways, making it difficult to breathe.

Although asthma is characterized by repeated attacks (during which symptoms progressively worsen), airway inflammation may persist even when symptoms are absent, and may therefore require long-term treatment with medication.

In people who develop asthma before age 30, attacks are more likely to be triggered by exposure to a specific environmental irritant, such as cigarette smoke, industrial fumes, pollen, mold, dust, animal dander or saliva, and perfumes. Exposure to irritants can trigger an asthma attack by causing the airways to "twitch" and narrow as they become plugged with sticky mucus.

In people who develop asthma after age 30, exercise, cold or

Some Drugs Can Worsen Asthma Symptoms

Make sure your doctor is aware of all the medications you're taking

Many older adults with asthma take a number of prescription and over-the-counter medications to treat a variety of conditions. Some of these medications may trigger or worsen asthma symptoms. If you take any of the medications discussed below, it's important to talk to your doctor about their possible negative effects on your asthma.

Medications That Interact With Asthma Drugs

It's not just prescription drugs that reduce the effectiveness of your asthma medications. You have to watch out for over-the-counter drugs, too.

Nonsteroidal anti-inflammatory drugs (NSAIDs). These over-the-counter pain relievers include aspirin, ibuprofen (Motrin, Advil), and naproxen (Naprosyn, Aleve). NSAIDS can trigger severe and even fatal asthma attacks. A safer over-the-counter alternative is acetaminophen (Tylenol). Alternative prescription painkillers include propoxyphone (Darvon), and codeine.

Beta-blockers. These prescription medications are given in pill form to treat conditions such as high blood pressure, heart disease, or migraines. Beta-blockers also come in the form of eye drops for treating glaucoma. Both forms of beta-blockers (see below) can worsen asthma symptoms by interfering with the effectiveness of beta-agonist asthma drugs.

There are 2 groups of beta-blockers: **non-specific,** which affect blood vessels and bronchial tissue, and **specific**, which affect blood vessels much more than bronchial tissue. Non-specific beta-blockers, such as propanalol (Inderal), are most likely to cause problems in people with asthma. Though specific beta-blockers, such as atenolol (Tenormin) or metoprolol (Lopressor), are less likely to cause problems in people with asthma, they still require close monitoring by your doctor.

ACE Inhibitors. These drugs are typically used to treat high blood pressure and heart disease. Lisinopril (Zestril) and enalopril (Vasotec) are examples. Although they usually don't make asthma worse, some people who use these drugs develop a very troublesome cough, which can trigger increased wheezing. In addition, any cough can lead to reflux (acid coming up from the stomach into the esophagus), which, in turn, can cause more cough and worsen asthma.

Diuretics. Diuretics, used to treat high blood pressure and congestive heart failure, help the body to excrete urine. Some diuretics can cause a loss in potassium and are therefore referred to as non-potassium-sparing diuretics. These diuretics may interact with asthma medications such as steroids and $beta_2$ agonists, which also lead to potassium loss. The result is an additive, dangerous amount of potassium depletion. If left untreated, this depletion increases the risk for disturbances in heart rhythm that can occasionally lead to cardiac arrest.

Non-potassium-sparing diuretics include thiazides—such as chlorothiazide (Diuril), chlorthalidone (Hygroton), indapamide (Lozol), and hydrochlorothiazide (Esidrix, HydroDiuril)—and loop diuretics, such as bumetanide (Bumex), furosemide (Lasix), and ethacrynic acid (Edecrin).

Sleeping pills and tranquilizers. Sleeping pills, tranquilizers, and other sedative drugs make you breathe more slowly and less deeply, which can be dangerous if you have lung problems such as asthma.

Asthma Drugs That Aggravate Other Health Conditions

Drug interactions are a 2-way street. In addition to some drugs worsening your asthma, some asthma drugs can aggravate other health conditions:

$Beta_2$ agonists and theophylline. Use of these asthma drugs should be monitored carefully because they can cause irregular heartbeats and worsen heart disease. If your doctor determines that it is too risky for you to rely solely on $beta_2$ agonists for your asthma treatment, he or she might recommend a combination inhaler with a short-acting $beta_2$ agonist and an anticholinergic drug (such as Combivent) as an alternative.

Theophylline. The dosage of theophylline may need to be reduced in some older patients with impaired liver function. Accumulation of theophylline in the bloodstream can lead to many side effects, some of which are serious, such as seizures, irregular heartbeat, and severe nausea and vomiting. Drugs that may increase theophylline blood levels include the acid reflux medication cimetidine (Tagamet) and antibiotics such as erythromycin and ciprofloxacin (Cipro). Drugs that may decrease theophylline blood levels include the anti-seizure drugs phenytoin (Dilantin) and carbamazepine (Tegretol).

Systemic corticosteroids. These drugs may aggravate congestive heart failure and lower the body's potassium levels, which can adversely affect the heart.

Corticosteroids. At high doses, corticosteroids may reduce bone mineral density and accelerate the development of osteoporosis.

Anticholinergics. Ipratropium bromide (Atrovent) and other anticholinergics can aggravate several pre-existing conditions, including glaucoma, an enlarged prostate, and obstruction of the neck of the bladder. ■

dry air, emotional stress, and gastroesophageal reflux (GERD) are more likely to trigger attacks (see "Asthma and Reflux," page 13).

Symptoms. The onset of an asthma attack may be gradual or sudden. Some attacks resolve on their own, but most require medication. Milder attacks are most common and usually begin with tightness in the chest and a cough. Wheezing may be heard with breathing. Restlessness and difficulty sleeping may accompany these symptoms. Sometimes these mild attacks seem to improve, only to be followed by the reappearance of persistent symptoms that may require treatment in a hospital.

During severe attacks, extreme shortness of breath is accompanied by wheezing, tightness in the chest, coughing up thick phlegm, sweating, a faster breathing rate, and a rapid pulse. Symptoms may last for only a few minutes, particularly if treated promptly, or may persist for hours or days, even after using medication. Coughing can continue for a week or longer after other acute symptoms disappear.

Diagnosis. Diagnosis during an attack is usually apparent from the symptoms, especially if the person has a history of asthma attacks. In older individuals, asthma must be distinguished from COPD and cardiac conditions such as heart failure or a heart attack. Heart failure can cause fluid to accumulate in the lungs, producing some of the same symptoms as asthma.

Between asthma attacks, a diagnosis may require pulmonary function tests to measure airway obstruction, an examination of mucus from the nose and lungs, and, possibly, allergy tests.

Prevention. People with asthma should avoid asthma triggers whenever possible and take preventive medications. A hand-held device called a peak flow meter measures how well air flows out of the lungs. Taking peak flow meter measurements at home is a simple and accurate way to detect a decline in lung function before symptoms begin. A person with asthma determines a "personal best" level of function—the highest flow rate consistently achieved when his or her asthma is under control. A person's personal best depends on gender, age, height, and other variables. Peak flow measurements that fall below this personal best level signal the need for more aggressive use of medications.

Treatment. People with asthma must have a plan of action in case of an attack. Inhaled medication should always be on hand for self-treatment. A severe attack requires taking medication immediately and quickly getting to a doctor's office or emergency room. A milder attack may require a call or visit to the doctor, if symptoms

Asthma and Reflux

What's the connection?

Up to 70% of people with asthma have gastroesophageal reflux disease (GERD), compared with 20–30% of the general population. These statistics suggest that if you have severe, chronic asthma which does not respond well to treatment, you are particularly susceptible to GERD.

What is GERD?

GERD is more than just heartburn, although that is the most common symptom. After you eat, a part of your digestive system called the lower esophageal sphincter normally stays closed as you digest food. But sometimes the sphincter relaxes, letting stomach acid flow back (reflux) into the esophagus.

In addition to heartburn, other symptoms of GERD include:

- Re-tasting your food after eating
- Difficulty or pain when swallowing
- Bad breath or sour taste
- Inflamed gums
- Excess saliva
- Chronic sore throat and laryngitis.

Some people with reflux have no symptoms, known as silent reflux.

If your GERD is not treated, it can lead to long-term health problems such as inflammation of the esophagus from stomach acid, which can cause bleeding or ulcers. Scars from tissue damage can narrow the esophagus and make swallowing difficult. In addition, some people develop a condition called Barrett's esophagus, in which cells in the esophageal lining become an abnormal shape and color, which over time can lead to cancer.

The GERD-Asthma Connection

Doctors are not sure exactly what the connection is between GERD and asthma, but there are several theories. If you have GERD, you may be breathing the digestive acid from the reflux into your lungs, where the acid irritates the lung's lining and causes spasms in the bronchi, resulting in an asthma attack. It is also possible that when acid enters your esophagus, it dissolves the lining and exposes segments of a major nerve that affects the lungs. This triggers a nerve reflex that makes your airways narrow to prevent acid from entering them, thereby causing shortness of breath.

You may have both GERD and asthma if you have:

- Increased asthma symptoms after you eat or exercise
- Increased asthma symptoms when you lie down
- Frequent coughing or hoarseness
- Asthma that doesn't respond to the standard asthma treatments.

Although the connection between GERD and asthma is not well understood, doctors have found that treating your GERD symptoms often relieves your asthma symptoms as well. On the other hand, certain asthma drugs may actually make your GERD worse. For example, bronchodilator medications may decrease lower esophageal sphincter pressure, making it easier for acid to back up. Theophylline, a commonly used bronchodilator, both increases the stomach's secretion of gastric acid and decreases lower esophageal sphincter pressure.

Diagnosis and Treatment

Your doctor may use a test called esophageal pH monitoring to diagnose GERD and determine how much reflux you have. The test involves placing a catheter through the nose, down the esophagus, and into the stomach to measure acid levels (pH) in the esophagus throughout the day.

If your doctor detects GERD, he or she may recommend esophageal and gastric endoscope, in which a tube with a tiny video camera is inserted through the mouth, down the esophagus and into the stomach to detect specific gastrointestinal problems that may be causing reflux symptoms. Your doctor may also search for *Helicobacter pylori* bacteria that thrive in the acidity of the stomach and have been linked to both GERD and peptic ulcers.

Medications

Over-the-counter antacids such as Tums, Rolaids, Maalox, Zantac, Tagamet, Pepsid, and Axed often relieve GERD, but if your symptoms persist for more than 2 weeks, talk to your doctor. He or she may recommend medications called proton pump inhibitors (such as Medium) that block or limit the amount of stomach acid your body produces. In rare circumstances, GERD may only be treatable through surgery.

Lifestyle Changes

You can make lifestyle changes to ease GERD symptoms:

- Sleep with your head elevated 6–8 inches. Gravity will help keep the stomach's contents in the stomach. Using extra pillows alone will not help. Place blocks of wood under the bedposts.
- Maintain a healthy weight.
- Don't smoke—smoking relaxes the lower esophageal sphincter.
- Drink less alcohol and caffeine—both relax the lower esophageal sphincter.
- Limit consumption of tomatoes and citrus fruits and juices, all of which are acidic and can irritate the esophagus.
- Eat smaller meals and avoid eating heavy meals at night.
- Don't lie down within 2–3 hours after eating.
- Wear loose belts and clothing to avoid pressure on the stomach. ■

persist longer than usual after using medication. Drug therapy includes bronchodilators and anti-inflammatory drugs. Bronchodilators reduce the constriction of airway (bronchial) muscles, while anti-inflammatory drugs help to overcome bronchial inflammation or excessive sensitivity to irritants.

Bronchodilators. Bronchodilators, which quickly open the airways by relaxing the bronchial muscles, are the fastest acting treatment for asthma attacks. They can be taken by mouth (in tablet or capsule form), but inhaled sprays ("inhalers") are usually preferred because oral forms take longer to act and may produce more side effects. Bronchodilators can be used as a preventive measure before exposure to triggers known to cause asthma attacks, such as exercise or cold air. In addition to helping prevent an attack or reducing the severity of an attack that does occur, bronchodilators can improve a person's ability to better tolerate such exposures.

The 3 types of bronchodilators are $beta_2$ agonists, anticholinergics, and methylxanthine derivatives. These drugs all work to keep airways open, but each does so in a different way. A person with asthma may therefore need more than one type of bronchodilator.

$Beta_2$ agonists are the most commonly used type of bronchodilator; they work the fastest and keep the airways open for many hours. The short-acting $beta_2$ drugs—albuterol (Proventil, Ventolin), levalbuterol (Xopenex), metaproterenol (Alupent), and pirbuterol (Maxair)—begin to act in about 10 minutes and last for 4–6 hours. Longer-acting $beta_2$ agents—salmeterol (Serevent) and formoterol (Foradil)—act within 15–30 minutes and continue to work for up to 12 hours.

If symptoms do not adequately improve, one option is to add either the anticholinergic ipratropium (Atrovent), which takes effect in 15–30 minutes and lasts 4–6 hours, or tiotropium powder inhaler (Spiriva HandiHaler), which involves inhaling 1 capsule every 24 hours. Combivent and Duoneb, which are combinations of the $beta_2$ agonist albuterol and the anticholinergic ipratropium, are also available. It is important to note that, when used excessively, $beta_2$ agonists can cause tremors and heart palpitations and can also become less effective (see feature on page 11).

People who cannot tolerate $beta_2$ agonists or anticholinergics, or who experience asthma symptoms at night, may benefit from one of the extended-release oral forms of the methylxanthine derivative theophylline (Theo-24,Theo-Dur,Uniphyl). Side effects of theophylline include nausea and insomnia.

Anti-inflammatory drugs. Continuous use of anti-inflammatory

NEW RESEARCH

Dry-Powder Inhalers Often Used Incorrectly

Dry-powder inhalers are used incorrectly just as frequently as older metered-dose inhalers, a new study of people with asthma and chronic obstructive pulmonary disease (COPD) reports.

Doctors have long been aware that metered-dose inhalers are often poorly used, but little information has been available about the use of newer dry powder inhalers. Researchers evaluated the inhalation technique of 1,404 people ages 15–88 who had either asthma or COPD. A trained observer recorded participants' inhalation techniques for each inhaler used, evaluating them against a step-by-step standardized checklist.

The study found that 24% of the participants used metered-dose inhalers incorrectly, but that only 3% used them incorrectly when they employed an add-on spacer device, which is designed to make using an inhaler easier. Among participants using the newer dry-powder inhalers, 17% used the Aerolizer Inhaler incorrectly, compared with 23% using the Turbuhaler and 24% using the Diskus.

The researchers concluded that adding a spacer device to a metered-dose inhaler, combined with proper training from a health care professional on how to use the inhaler, is the best strategy for minimizing poor inhalation techniques (and is better than simply switching to a dry-powder inhaler).

ANNALS OF ALLERGY, ASTHMA AND IMMUNOLOGY
Volume 93, page 439
November 2004

drugs to control chronic inflammation is a critical component of asthma therapy in people with frequent symptoms (people with mild asthma are generally not treated with anti-inflammatory drugs). The first choice of medications to counteract inflammation in adults is inhaled corticosteroids, which include beclomethasone (Beclovent, Vanceril, QVAR); triamcinolone (Azmacort); budesonide (Pulmicort); flunisolide (AeroBid); and fluticasone (Flovent). A combination of the corticosteroid fluticasone and the long-acting $beta_2$ agonist salmeterol are also available (Advair). The most frequent side effects of inhaled corticosteroids are irritation of the throat and yeast infection in the mouth and throat. These side effects can be reduced by rinsing the mouth (by swishing water around in the mouth, gently gargling, and spitting out the water) and cleaning the inhaler after each use.

When used for long periods of time, corticosteroids can cause osteoporosis (bone loss), high blood pressure, roundness of the face, weight gain, diabetes, cataracts, and thinning of the skin; these side effects are less common with inhaled corticosteroids, as little of the medication is absorbed into the bloodstream.

Oral corticosteroids, such as methylprednisolone (Medrol) and prednisone (Deltasone, Sterapred), take 6 hours to start working and must be used at the lowest effective dose and for the shortest time possible to avoid side effects. Using oral corticosteroids for more than a few weeks suppresses the adrenal gland—hormones produced by the adrenal gland are critical for maintaining the body's normal functions. If used for prolonged periods, the medications must be discontinued slowly to allow recovery of adrenal function.

Inhaled nonsteroidal anti-inflammatory drugs (NSAIDs) can also used in the treatment of asthma. Cromolyn (Intal) and nedocromil (Tilade), which work by preventing the release of histamine, are inhaled drugs used only for long-term prevention of asthma symptoms (not for immediate relief). The leukotriene modifiers montelukast (Singulair), zafirlukast (Accolate), and zileuton (Zyflo), which counteract the actions of leukotrienes (cell products that narrow the airways and stimulate the production of mucus), help prevent exercise-induced asthma, and can enhance the action of inhaled corticosteroids; however, the effectiveness of these medications varies considerably from person to person.

Inhaled medications are usually administered through a device called a metered dose inhaler (MDI). An MDI delivers a highly concentrated amount of medication directly to the airways. Inhaled medications are less likely to produce systemic (affecting

NEW RESEARCH

Pet Removal May Allow Asthmatics to Reduce Corticosteroid Dosage

Removing pets from the homes of people with allergic asthma, combined with drug treatment, reduces airway "twitchiness" more than medication alone in people whose asthma is triggered by pet dander, a new study finds. Pet removal also enabled patients to reduce their dosage of inhaled corticosteroids.

Researchers studied 20 people with pet allergic asthma who owned pets such as hamsters, cats, dogs, and ferrets. Half the participants removed their pets; half did not. All participants were treated with inhaled corticosteroids or other medications (as needed), according to the severity of their asthma. Before and after starting medication, the participants underwent testing to determine the sensitivity of their airways and to detect problems with their breathing.

A year later, the people who removed their pets had a much greater reduction in the tendency of their airways to constrict and cause breathing problems, compared with the people who kept their pets. None of those who gave away their pets needed inhaled steroid therapy, compared with 9 of the 10 who kept their pets.

Because many pet owners will not consider removing their pets, studies that directly compare pet removal with other strategies, such as air purification, use of hypoallergenic products, and smoking cessation, are needed.

CHEST
Volume 127, page 1565
May 2005

Commonly Used Bronchodilators 2006

Drug Type	Drug Class	Generic Name	Brand Name
Inhaled	Anticholinergics, short-acting	ipratropium, standard inhaler	Atrovent
	Anticholinergics, long-acting	tiotropium, powder inhaler	Spiriva HandiHaler
	$Beta_2$ agonists, short-acting	albuterol, standard inhaler	Proventil
		albuterol, non-CFC inhaler	Proventil HFA Ventolin HFA
		metaproterenol, standard inhaler	Alupent
		pirbuterol, standard inhaler	Maxair
	$Beta_2$ agonists, long-acting	salmeterol, powder inhaler	Serevent Diskus
		formoterol, powder inhaler	Foradil Aerolizer
	Combination agents	albuterol and ipratropium, standard inhaler	Combivent
		albuterol and ipratropium, nebulizer	DuoNeb
		salmeterol and fluticasone, powder inhaler	Advair Diskus

* These dosages represent an average range for the treatment of asthma and chronic obstructive pulmonary disease. The precise effective dosage varies from patient to patient and depends on many factors. Do not make any changes in your medication without consulting your doctor.

Average Daily Dosage*	Possible Side Effects
2 puffs every 4–6 hours 1 capsule inhaled every 24 hours	Common side effects include dry mouth, cough, and unpleasant taste. Rare but serious side effects include persistent constipation, lower abdominal pain or bloating, wheezing or difficulty breathing, tightness in chest, severe eye pain, skin rash or hives, and swelling of the face, lips, or eyelids.
2 puffs every 4–6 hours 2 puffs every 4–6 hours	Common side effects include nervousness, tremor, dizziness, headache, and insomnia. Rare but serious side effects include severe breathing difficulty (signs include persistent wheezing, coughing, shortness of breath, confusion, bluish color to lips or fingernails, and inability to speak).
2–3 puffs every 3–4 hours	Common side effects include trouble sleeping, dry mouth, sore throat, nervousness, and restlessness. Rare but serious side effects include severe breathing difficulty (signs include persistent wheezing, coughing, shortness of breath, confusion, bluish color to lips or fingernails, and inability to speak).
1–2 puffs every 4–6 hours	Common side effects include sleeping difficulty, dry mouth, sore throat, nervousness, excitability, and restlessness. Rare but serious side effects include severe breathing difficulty (signs include persistent wheezing, coughing, shortness of breath, confusion, bluish color to lips or fingernails, and inability to speak), chest pain or heaviness, irregular heartbeat, light-headedness, fainting, severe weakness, and severe headaches.
1 inhalation 2 times a day	Common side effects include headache, sore throat, and runny or stuffy nose. Rare but serious side effects include severe breathing difficulty (signs include persistent wheezing, coughing, shortness of breath, confusion, bluish color to lips or fingernails, and inability to speak), chest pain or heaviness, irregular heartbeat, light-headedness, fainting, severe weakness, and severe headache.
1– 2 inhalations 2 times a day	Common side effects include fast heartbeat, headache, nervousness, and trembling. Rare but serious side effects include shortness of breath, difficulty breathing, tightness in the chest, increased wheezing, swelling of the face or eyelids, and skin rash or hives.
2 inhalation 4 times a day	Common side effects include coughing, headache, and nausea. Rare but serious side effects include increased wheezing, shortness of breath, chest pain, irregular heartbeat, skin rash or hives, and swelling of the face, lips, eyelids, mouth, or throat.
1 vial 4–6 times a day	There are no common side effects. Rare but serious side effects include swelling of the face, lips, eyelids, mouth, or throat, shortness of breath, increased wheezing, chest pain or discomfort, irregular heartbeat, skin rash or hives, coughing, headache, and nausea.
1 puff 2 times a day	Common side effects include a high-pitched noise while breathing, body aches, runny or stuffy nose, coughing, dry or sore throat, fever, hoarseness, swollen glands, trouble swallowing, voice changes, and sneezing. Rare but serious side effects include difficulty breathing; shortness of breath; tightness in the chest; increased wheezing; black, tarry stools; chest pain; chills; painful or difficult urination; ulcers; white spots on lips or mouth; fatigue; burning, tingling, or numb sensation in hands and feet; abdominal pain; loss of appetite; nausea; and flu-like symptoms.

Commonly Used Bronchodilators 2006—continued

Drug Type	Drug Class	Generic Name	Brand Name
Oral	Methylxanthine derivatives	theophylline, extended-release capsule, 24 hr	Theo-24
		theophylline, extended-release tablet, 12 hr	Theo-Dur
		theophylline, extended-release tablet, 24 hr	Uniphyl

* These dosages represent an average range for the treatment of asthma and chronic obstructive pulmonary disease. The precise effective dosage varies from patient to patient and depends on many factors. Do not make any changes in your medication without consulting your doctor.

the whole body) side effects than oral medications. Proper technique is important, and many people use their MDI incorrectly. (See "Using a Metered Dose Inhaler" on page 20.) People who find it difficult to use an MDI can add a spacer—an attachment that eliminates the need to release the medication and inhale simultaneously. Another option is to use a device called a nebulizer, which vaporizes liquid medication into a fine mist that can be inhaled easily.

Monoclonal antibody. If inhaled corticosteroids do not adequately control severe allergy-related asthma, people aged 12 years and older may benefit from omalizumab (Xolair), a medication approved in 2003. Omalizumab, which is injected once or twice a month, decreases the body's immune response to inhaled allergens (such as dust mites or animal dander) by blocking the antibody IgE. The annual cost of treatment, however, is between $5,000 and $10,000.

Chronic Obstructive Pulmonary Disease (COPD)

Chronic obstructive pulmonary disease is a term that encompasses chronic bronchitis and emphysema. The symptoms of COPD develop slowly over several years and include wheezing, a chronic cough that produces phlegm, and progressive shortness of breath. COPD is the fourth leading cause of death in the United States.

Emphysema is a disorder characterized by destruction of lung tissue, including its elastic fibers. By reducing the elasticity of the lungs and destroying the walls between the air sacs, emphysema

Average Daily Dosage*	Possible Side Effects
300–600 mg	Common side effects include restlessness, insomnia, loss of appetite, nervousness, irritability, and nausea. Rare but serious side effects include vomiting; trembling; confusion; rapid, irregular, or pounding pulse; chest pain; dizziness; convulsions; and skin rash.
300–600 mg	
300–600 mg	

leads to the collapse of the airways, reducing airflow. More than 3 million Americans have emphysema, and more than 15,000 people die of it each year. Emphysema rates are highest among men age 65 years and older. You might remember that Johnny Carson died of the disease last year.

Chronic bronchitis is a recurrent problem defined by coughing up phlegm nearly every day for at least three months of the year (for example, every winter) for 2 or more consecutive years. The condition reduces the width of the airways through a combination of airway inflammation and overproduction of mucus. There are more than 9 million cases of chronic bronchitis a year in the U.S. and more than 1,000 deaths. Chronic bronchitis is more prevalent in women than in men.

Causes. Cigarette smoking causes the vast majority of COPD cases. Cigarette smoke is thought to release enzymes that damage a protein called elastin, which makes the lungs elastic. Smoking is also believed to inactivate $alpha_1$ antitrypsin, a protein produced by the liver that normally protects elastin from the action of these enzymes.

About 1 in 2,500 people worldwide has a genetic defect that prevents the secretion of $alpha_1$ antitrypsin by the liver and increases the risk of developing premature emphysema, especially in smokers. Other factors that raise a person's risk of emphysema include a family history of COPD, male gender, respiratory illnesses in childhood, and work-related exposure to pollutants.

Using a Metered Dose Inhaler

Getting medicine to your lungs

For people with asthma or chronic obstructive pulmonary disease (COPD), using an inhaler is the fastest method of delivering medication to the lungs. It is also the safest; the risk of side effects is lower than with tablets or capsules because inhaled medications act primarily on the lungs.

Inhaled medications may be delivered 3 ways—the most common is using a metered dose inhaler (MDI), a pressurized canister that releases an aerosol spray. Dry powder inhalers (such as Diskhaler and Turbuhaler) and nebulizers are the other 2 options for delivering inhaled medications to the lungs.

An inhaler can be difficult to use because it requires coordination between releasing the medication and breathing in. Even when an inhaler is used correctly, most of the medication sticks to the back of the throat and no more than 10%–20% reaches the lungs. The key to getting the most from your inhaler is to use the proper technique. If you follow these steps on how to use an MDI, more of the medicine will reach your lungs. In addition, your doctor can observe you using your inhaler to make sure that you are using it properly.

Using a Metered Dose Inhaler

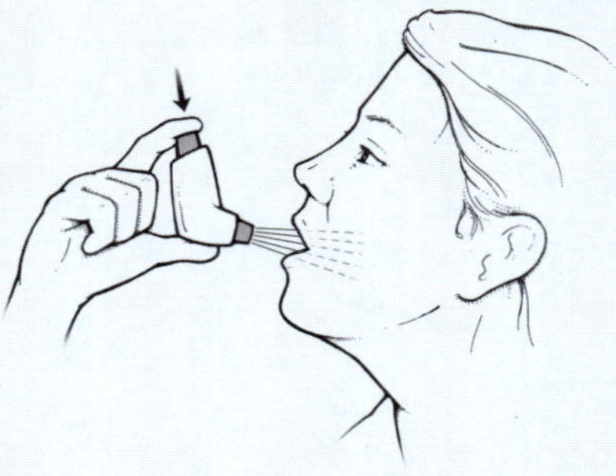

1. Place the metal canister into the plastic mouthpiece.

2. Remove the cap from the mouthpiece and shake the inhaler for 5–10 seconds.

3. Breathe out to the end of a normal breath (but don't force air out).

4. Hold the mouthpiece of the inhaler 1–2 inches (about 2 finger widths) from your mouth, tilt your head back slightly, and open your mouth wide. Start to breathe in slowly as you press down once on the metal canister to release a puff of medication.

5. Continue to inhale until your lungs are full (for about 5 seconds). Inhaling too quickly will increase the amount of medication that sticks to the back of the throat.

6. Hold your breath for 10 seconds, or for as long as is comfortable.

7. Before exhaling, move the inhaler away from your mouth and release your finger from the canister.

8. Replace the cap on the mouthpiece to avoid contamination by dust and other particles.

9. For an additional dose, wait 1 minute and repeat steps 2–8.

10. Clean the plastic mouthpiece once a week by removing the metal canister and rinsing the plastic portion in warm water; allow it to air dry. Replace the metal canister and the cap on the mouthpiece.

When Using a Spacer

A spacer (also called a holding chamber) holds the medication for a few seconds after it has been released from the inhaler. This delay can be helpful for people who have difficulty coordinating their breathing with the use of an inhaler. You may also benefit from a spacer because they help reduce side effects such as sore throat and hoarseness caused by medication sticking to the back of the throat.

Spacers are simple to use, can be fitted to most inhalers and can either be rigid or collapsible. Here are guidelines for both types of spacers:

Symptoms. People who develop COPD typically began smoking at an early age and have a long history of a morning cough that produces phlegm. Lung function often declines slowly over many years. Most people only seek medical advice after noticing significant shortness of breath on exertion, which typically starts only after age 50. As COPD worsens, breathlessness begins to severely limit activities.

Although lung function tends to decrease slowly, the decline is often punctuated by acute episodes of worsening symptoms, usually due to a viral or bacterial infection. These acute episodes are marked by increased shortness of breath, wheezing, and a cough that produces greater than usual amounts of phlegm. Though

Using a Rigid Spacer

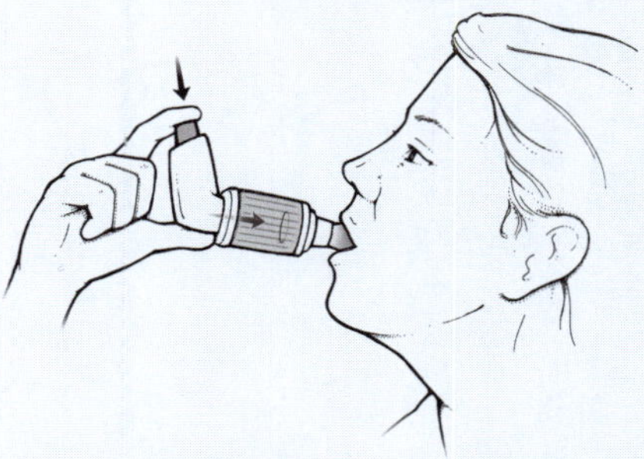

Press down on the metal canister so that the spacer fills with medication.

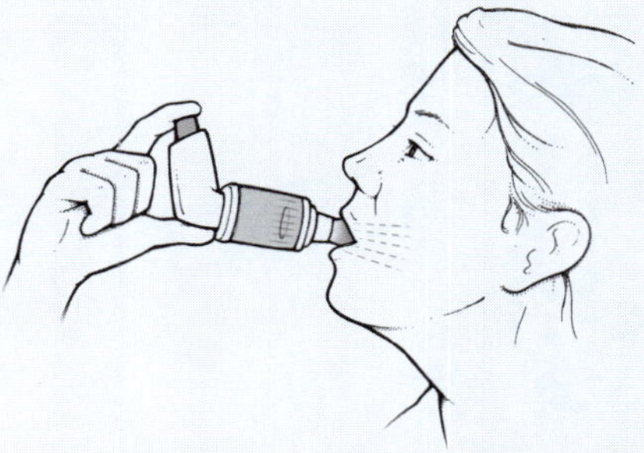

Breathe in slowly for about 5 seconds.

1. Remove the cap from the mouthpiece of the inhaler and insert the mouthpiece into the large opening of the rigid spacer. For a collapsible spacer, insert the mouthpiece of the spacer into the opening of the reservoir bag. Align the locking tabs and twist to lock. Then, untwist the reservoir bag until it is entirely open.

2. For a rigid spacer, hold the spacer and inhaler together and shake for 5–10 seconds. For a collapsible spacer, shake the metal canister separately for 5 seconds before inserting it into the adapter port of the spacer's mouthpiece.

3. Breathe out, then put the mouthpiece in your mouth, closing your lips around it.

4. Press the metal canister down.

5. Breathe in slowly for about 5 seconds.

6. Hold your breath for about 10 seconds or as long as is comfortable.

7. If your spacer is rigid, slowly exhale through your mouth or nose (not into the spacer), then take another breath through the mouthpiece to ensure you receive the full amount of medication released by the inhaler. If you have a collapsible spacer, slowly exhale into the spacer. Breathe in and out a second time (steps 5 and 6) with your lips around the mouthpiece.

8. Repeat steps 2–7 for each puff that your doctor prescribes, waiting a full minute between each.

9. To ensure that your spacer is clean, run warm water through the large opening and allow it to air dry. If your spacer is collapsible you should replace it once or twice each month. ■

Using a Collapsible Spacer

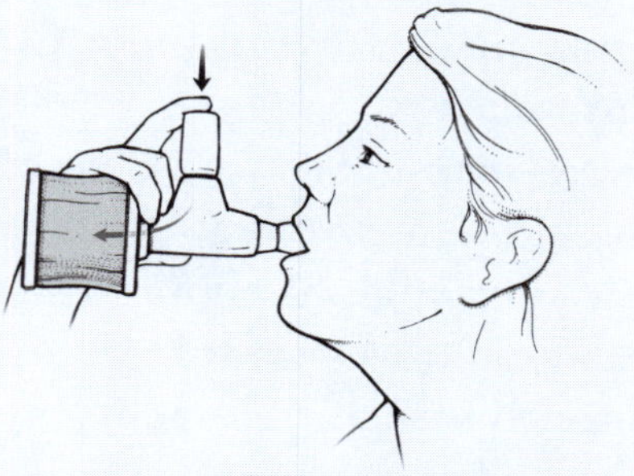

Press down on the metal canister so that the spacer fills with medication.

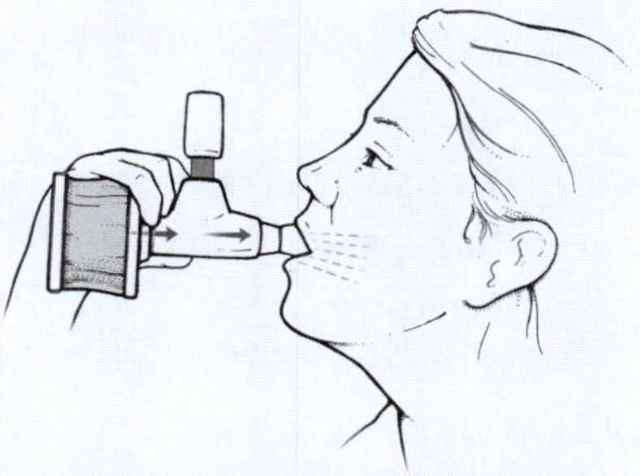

Breathe in slowly for about five seconds.

acute episodes may be severe enough to be life threatening, they do not necessarily speed the rate of disease progression. COPD may also cause low levels of oxygen in the blood, which can lead to pulmonary hypertension, a rise in pressure in the arteries to the lungs. Pulmonary hypertension increases the workload of the heart's right ventricle (the lower chamber of the heart), causing it to enlarge. At advanced stages of COPD, patients often become thin because they find eating tiring, and because the work of breathing burns more calories than it does in healthy people.

Diagnosis. Your doctor will perform a physical exam and listen to the breath sounds with a stethoscope. He or she will also look at the results of spirometry testing; people with COPD have abnormal results. Spirometry testing not only indicates the presence and severity of COPD but also helps define the prognosis.

Imaging tests are also used for diagnosis. A chest x-ray may show increased volume of air in the lungs and enlargement of the central pulmonary artery, which extends from the heart's right ventricle to the lungs. In addition, changes can sometimes be seen on an electrocardiogram (EKG, a non-invasive test that records the electrical activity of the heart) depending on the stage of the disease.

Seeking a genetic cause by measuring levels of $alpha_1$ antitrypsin may be useful when COPD occurs in a young person or a nonsmoker.

Prevention. Steering clear of cigarette smoking is the most obvious and effective way to prevent COPD. Some people with a deficiency of $alpha_1$ antitrypsin may receive some protection from weekly or twice-monthly intravenous (I.V.) injections of the substance, but such treatments are expensive, inconvenient, and not always effective.

Treatment. Only about half of people with COPD survive for 10 years or more after the diagnosis is made. The goals of COPD treatment are not only to prolong life, but to help maintain independence and alleviate discomfort. These goals are achieved through a combination of lifestyle modifications, medications, vaccinations, oxygen therapy, and, occasionally, surgical procedures.

Lifestyle modifications. The 2 interventions associated with improved survival in people with COPD are smoking cessation and supplemental oxygen. Even people with advanced COPD can increase their life expectancy if they stop smoking. Avoiding exposure to other airborne toxins (including secondhand cigarette smoke), exercising as much as possible, and following an adequate diet are also important. If eating is tiring, consuming several small meals a day rather than a few large ones is often helpful. Adding a liquid protein supplement to the daily diet can improve overall nutrition and help prevent weight loss. It is also essential to drink plenty of fluids to avoid dehydration. If you have COPD, you should not push yourself when you get tired, and you should avoid exerting yourself when it is too hot, too cold, humid, or when air quality is poor.

Even routine tasks can be exhausting when you have severe COPD. Activities such as bathing, grooming, and dressing often require a great deal of effort, but careful planning can help conserve energy, allowing many people to get through these tasks more quickly and easily.

Plan to bathe, groom, and dress at times when you're feeling most energetic. Also, gather all the supplies you will need before you start. When bathing, instead of standing in the shower, use a bath stool or take baths. Because excess humidity can make it tougher to breathe, use warm water rather than hot, leave the bathroom door open, turn on exhaust fans, and open a window whenever possible. Use a long-handled brush or sponge to avoid stretching to wash your back and feet. Oxygen can still be used in the tub or shower—just drape the tube over the shower rod or side of the tub. (It's safe to remove the nasal cannula briefly while washing your face.) Instead of using a towel to dry off, try wearing a long terrycloth robe. Or try blotting rather than rubbing with the towel to dry yourself; it takes less effort.

To make grooming easier, choose a simple hairstyle that doesn't require extensive blow-drying or styling. Conserve energy by sitting in front of a low mirror when shaving or applying makeup, rather than standing bent over the bathroom sink. Avoid products that are aerosolized or heavily scented, which may irritate the lungs. Most deodorants are available in roll-on or solid formulations, and many are also fragrance-free. Perfumes and colognes can make it more difficult to breathe, so avoid using these products.

To simplify the daily dressing routine, store clothes—especially those worn frequently—in places that don't require bending or reaching. Avoid tight-fitting clothing that can make breathing difficult. For example, men can wear suspenders instead of belts, and women can wear camisoles or sports bras instead of regular bras. Don't wear socks or stockings with elastic bands, since they can restrict circulation. (Support hosiery recommended by your doctor is the exception.) Slip-on shoes mean you don't have to bend over to tie shoelaces. A long shoehorn (12–18 inches) can make it easier to put shoes on. To conserve energy, stay seated as long as possible while dressing, and dress your lower half first, as it is usually more difficult. Putting your underwear inside your pants and pulling both on together may be helpful as well.

Pulmonary rehabilitation programs can be very beneficial for many people with COPD. Pulmonary rehabilitation is a comprehensive preventive health care program provided by a team of health professionals to help people cope physically, psychologically, and socially with COPD. A typical rehabilitation program focuses on breathing exercises, exercise reconditioning, progressive relaxation training, stress and panic control techniques, smoking cessation, and educational programs on medication, diet, exercise, and

NEW RESEARCH

Some Beta-Blockers May Have Negative Effects in COPD Patients

Some beta-blockers used to treat hypertension, heart disease, and migraines may have detrimental effects on the lungs of people with chronic obstructive pulmonary disease (COPD), a new study suggests.

Researchers gave 15 COPD patients propranolol (Inderal), metoprolol (Lopressor, Toprol XL), celiprolol (another beta blocker which is not available in the U.S.), or a placebo for 4 days, followed by 3 days of no beta-blockers. On the fourth day of treatment, the patients' lung function was measured. They were then given formoterol (Foradil), a long-acting beta-agonist, which counters the effects of beta-blockers by stimulating beta-receptors rather than blocking them. Lung function was measured again.

The researchers found that patients treated with propranolol had noticeably decreased lung function and that their lung function improved more slowly after inhalation of the beta-agonist drug. Both propranolol and metoprolol also increased airway hyper-sensitivity.

In people with COPD, doctors and patients should be aware that different types of beta-blockers may have different effects on the lungs. The anticipated beneficial cardiovascular effects of a beta-blocker must be weighed against the potential detrimental effects on the lungs.

CHEST
Volume 127, page 818
March 2005

Commonly Used Asthma and COPD Anti-Inflammatory Drugs 2006

Drug Type	Drug Class	Generic Name	Brand Name
Inhaled	Corticosteroids, long-acting	budesonide, powder inhaler	Pulmicort Turbuhaler
		flunisolide, standard inhaler	AeroBid
		flunisolide, menthol, standard inhaler	AeroBid-M
		fluticasone, powder inhaler	Flovent
		fluticasone, powder inhaler	Flovent Rotadisk
	Corticosteroids, short-acting	beclomethasone, standard inhaler	Vanceril
		triamcinolone, standard inhaler	Azmacort
	Respiratory inhalers, nonsteroidal	cromolyn, standard inhaler	Intal
		nedocromil, standard inhaler	Tilade
Oral	Corticosteroids, short-acting	methylprednisolone	Medrol
		prednisone	Deltasone Sterapred
	Leukotriene modifiers, nonsteroidal	montelukast	Singulair
		zafirlukast	Accolate
		zileuton	Zyflo

* These dosages represent an average range for the treatment. The precise effective dosage varies from patient to patient and depends on many factors. Do not make any changes in your medication without consulting your doctor.

Average Daily Dosage*	Possible Side Effects
1–2 puffs 2 times a day 2 puffs 2 times a day 2 puffs 2 times a day 1–2 puffs 2 times a day 1–2 puffs 2 times a day	Side effects are not common, but can include a dry or irritated mouth or throat, cough, and hoarseness. Contact your doctor if these side effects are severe, or if you develop white spots or sores in your mouth.
2 puffs 3–4 times a day 2 puffs 3–4 times a day or 4 puffs 2 times a day	Side effects are not common, but can include a dry or irritated mouth or throat, cough, and hoarseness. Contact your doctor if these side effects are severe, or if you develop white spots or sores in your mouth.
2 puffs 4 times a day	Common side effects include throat irritation and dryness. Rare but serious side effects include difficulty swallowing; hives; itching; swelling of the face, lips, or eyelids; rash; and nosebleeds.
2 puffs 4 times a day	There are no common side effects. Rare but serious side effects include increased wheezing, tightness or pain in the chest, and difficulty breathing.
4–160 mg 5–100 mg	Common side effects include increased appetite, indigestion, nervousness, insomnia, greater susceptibility to infections, increased blood pressure, slowed wound healing, weight gain, easy bruising, and fluid retention. Rare but serious side effects include vision problems, frequent urination, increased thirst, rectal bleeding, blistering skin, confusion, hallucinations, paranoia, euphoria, depression, and mood swings.
10 mg	Common side effects include headache. Rare but serious side effects include skin rash (indicating potentially life-threatening allergic reaction) and gastroenteritis (causing loss of appetite, nausea, vomiting, stomach upset, fever, and diarrhea).
40 mg	Common side effects include headache. Rare but serious side effects include burning or prickling sensation, skin rash, and liver dysfunction (symptoms include abdominal pain, nausea, fatigue, lethargy, itching, yellow discoloration of the eyes or skin, and flu-like symptoms).
2,400 mg	Common side effects include headache, general pain, abdominal pain, nausea, indigestion, muscle soreness, and weakness. Rare but serious side effects include liver problems causing nausea, fatigue, lethargy, skin rash or itching, yellow discoloration of the eyes or skin, flu-like symptoms, and urine that is unusually dark.

caring for and operating respiratory therapy equipment.

Breath training is an important part of pulmonary rehabilitation. The objective is to help a person control his or her breathing rate, decrease the amount of energy required for breathing, and improve the position and function of the respiratory muscles. A respiratory therapist can help people with COPD practice the following techniques:

- **Pursed-lip breathing.** Inhale through your nose, then exhale with your lips pursed in a whistling or kissing position. Each inhalation should take about 2 seconds, and each exhalation should last about 4–6 seconds. It is not clear how pursed-lip breathing brings symptom relief, but it appears to work by keeping the airways open.
- **Diaphragmatic breathing.** The diaphragm is the main muscle used for normal breathing. People with COPD, however, may also use the muscles in the rib cage, neck, and abdomen to breathe. This method is less efficient than using the diaphragm. To practice using the diaphragm, lie on your back, place your hand or a small book on your abdomen, and breathe. Your hand or the book should rise on inhalation and fall on exhalation. Practice for 20 minutes twice daily. Once you have mastered this skill while lying down, try to do it while sitting up (without the book, of course).
- **Forward-bending posture.** Breathing while bending slightly forward from the waist relieves symptoms for some people with severe COPD, possibly because the diaphragm has more room to expand. Some research suggests that pulmonary rehabilitation can increase survival, but this has not been proven.

Medications. Despite their fixed lung obstruction, many people with COPD also have some reversible airway obstruction that may respond somewhat to bronchodilators. The $beta_2$ agonists and anticholinergics, which are described on page 14, are used most commonly. The methylxanthine derivative theophylline is less effective than $beta_2$ agonists, but it eases symptoms in about 20% of people with COPD.

If bronchodilators fail to relieve airway obstruction adequately, corticosteroids (both oral and inhaled; described on page 15) may diminish inflammation in some people. However, corticosteroids are less effective for COPD than for asthma, and their side effects may be more severe in older people. Because of the difficulty in predicting who will respond to corticosteroid therapy, a carefully monitored 2–3 week trial period of oral corticosteroids is often conducted. Oral corticosteroids are discontinued immediately in people who do not benefit from them. In people who do show improvement, the medications are tapered to the lowest possible effective dose. Inhaled corticosteroids may be helpful in some people, and their role in the treatment of COPD is being evaluated.

Expectorants (such as guaifenesin, found in Robitussin and other medications) may help to loosen mucus secretions in the airways. Antibiotics (such as tetracycline, ampicillin, erythromycin, and combinations of trimethoprim and sulfamethoxazole) are prescribed when increased production of yellow or green phlegm signals a respiratory infection that can aggravate COPD. Although moderate worsening of symptoms can be treated at home, severe episodes require hospitalization.

Mucus clearance devices. People with COPD who have chronic, moderate-to-severe mucus accumulation may benefit from a mucus clearance device—a small handheld device shaped like a pipe. Blowing into it creates vibrations in the chest that loosen mucus and help medication penetrate the lungs more easily. Some studies suggest that using a mucus clearance device before an inhaled bronchodilator can improve both lung function and exercise capacity, while reducing shortness of breath.

Vaccinations. People with COPD should have annual flu shots as well as a pneumonia vaccine about once every 6 years to minimize the risk of infections that can lead to episodes of temporary but severely worsened symptoms.

Oxygen therapy. Some people with COPD benefit not only from breath exercises, improved breathing technique, and medications, but also from home oxygen therapy. Home oxygen therapy typically enhances sleep and mood, increases mental alertness and stamina, allows people to carry out daily activities more efficiently, and may prevent the development of cor pulmonale (heart disease caused by high blood pressure in the lungs) by reducing the blood pressure in the lungs and the workload of the right side of the heart.

To determine if a person needs oxygen therapy, your doctor will measure oxygen levels in the blood (along with other variables such as carbon dioxide levels). Having too little oxygen in the blood can cause symptoms such as fatigue, irritability, an inability to concentrate, breathlessness, heart problems, and fluid retention.

If oxygen therapy is recommended, your doctor will write a prescription detailing the flow rate (how many liters of oxygen breathed in per minute). Different flow rates may be prescribed for different activities, such as sleeping versus exercising. Using too

NEW RESEARCH

Non-Smoking Women Whose Husbands Smoke Have Increased Risk of Stroke

Women who don't smoke—but live with men who do—have an increased risk of stroke, a new study reports. The risk increases with the number of cigarettes and the length of time their husbands have smoked.

The study included 60,377 women from the Shanghai Women's Health Study, aged 40–70 years. Interviewers asked the women about their history of diagnosed stroke and their husbands' smoking habits. Of the women, 526 had a history of stroke; risk rose with the daily number of cigarettes and length of time their husbands smoked. Women whose husbands were smoking 1–9 cigarettes a day had a 28% higher risk of stroke; those whose husbands smoked 10–19 cigarettes a day had a 32% higher risk of stroke; and those whose husbands smoked 20 or more cigarettes a day had a 62% higher risk of stroke.

The effects of secondhand smoke on women is easier to study in China than in other countries because two-thirds of men but few women smoke. In addition, the high rate of stable marriage in China facilitates investigating the effects of long-term secondhand smoke exposure on female nonsmokers.

AMERICAN JOURNAL OF EPIDEMIOLOGY
Volume 161, page 213
February 1, 2005

Travel and Oxygen

Planning ahead is key

These days, it's possible for people who use supplemental oxygen to travel by just about any mode of transportation. For a big trip to go smoothly, though, you'll need to do some advance planning in conjunction with your doctor and oxygen supplier. If you are visiting a destination at a high altitude, such as Denver, you may need to have your oxygen flow rate adjusted, or you may need supplemental oxygen even if you don't normally use it at home. Be sure to mention your destination to your doctor.

By Air

Call your doctor as soon as you know you're going away. If you have COPD and don't normally use supplemental oxygen, you may now need it if you're traveling by air, as low oxygen levels in the airplane cabin may adversely affect your breathing. Your doctor will give you a pre-flight assessment, including measurement of your blood oxygen level and general lung function tests. Based on the assessment, your doctor may recommend the use of in-flight oxygen. If you already are on supplemental oxygen, your doctor may recommend increasing the oxygen flow rate during the flight.

If you do need in-flight oxygen, you will need a letter on your doctor's letterhead with his or her name and contact information, information about your lung disorder, approval for air travel and verification of need for in-flight oxygen, and information about the oxygen flow rate in liters per minute and duration of use. Bring a copy for each flight you'll be on.

Also, ask your doctor for prescriptions for your medications, which you should carry onboard in case your luggage is lost or delayed. Your doctor may give you a supply of certain medications for emergencies, such as antibiotics to use if you develop a bacterial lung infection. These, too, should be in your carry-on bag, not in checked luggage.

Notify the airline at least 72 hours before the trip. Until last year, the Federal Aviation Administration (FAA) did not allow travelers to carry their own oxygen supply aboard commercial aircraft. But starting in August 2005, a new FAA rule allows passengers who require medical oxygen to take certain portable oxygen concentrators on board. The allowable concentrators are made by AirSept Corporation and Inogen Inc. The FAA permits the devices to be used throughout the flight, including takeoff and landing.

Passengers using concentrators during a flight are required to inform the pilot that they are doing so and provide a written statement signed by a licensed physician that verifies the passenger's ability to use the device.

It's important to note that the FAA regulation does not require individual airlines to let passengers use oxygen concentrators (it allows each airline to make its own policy). You should therefore make arrangements directly with the airline. Some airlines require at least 72 hours advance notice, particularly for international flights. It's a good idea to reconfirm your oxygen arrangements before your trip and to arrive at the airport early.

Ask what the airline charges for supplying in-flight oxygen. Do they charge for each flight? Check to see if your medical insurance will

much oxygen in some patients can slow breathing, allowing carbon dioxide to build up in the blood, so it's important to carefully follow the flow rates determined by your doctor.

People with COPD who need and use continuous oxygen therapy 24 hours a day appear to have a longer life span than those who use it only while awake (15 hours per day); in turn, people who use oxygen therapy 15 hours per day do better than people who use it only while sleeping.

Home oxygen therapy equipment. A variety of oxygen delivery systems and oxygen concentration devices are available. All forms of oxygen therapy are expensive; costs may be several hundred dollars a month, depending on the type of system. Oxygen concentrators are the least costly, although their use can increase your electric bill.

cover the costs of in-flight oxygen.

Ask whether you can bring your own empty oxygen equipment. Some airlines will allow you to bring empty personal oxygen equipment onboard or check it with your baggage. Ask if you will be able to bring your own cannula or mask; if not, find out whether the airline will provide one or both of these.

Ask about seat requirements. Some airlines may require you to buy an additional seat if you will need more than a certain number of oxygen cylinders.

Make arrangements for oxygen at layover stops. Airlines do not make arrangements for oxygen on the ground, so you'll need to ask your doctor and oxygen supplier to help you make arrangements. If at all possible, try to arrange for direct flights to avoid this problem.

Call an oxygen supplier in your destination city ahead of time. Your oxygen supplier can help make sure you have a supply of oxygen waiting for you when you arrive. Oxygen is widely available in Europe and Japan. When traveling abroad, be sure to have the right electrical version adapters for your equipment. You may also need liquid oxygen adapters with metric threads.

Before getting onboard, check the equipment. Make sure the oxygen cylinders are full, the equipment is working properly, and the flow meter has been set to the proper liter flow per minute.

By Car

When planning your trip, figure out your route and where you will stop to refill your oxygen tank. Ask your oxygen supplier for help in contacting local suppliers and arranging for them to have your oxygen ready when you get there.

Store oxygen upright, away from heat. Don't put oxygen in the trunk, where it can overheat. Because oxygen containers release small amounts of gas, keep a window partially open, no matter what the weather.

Plan for frequent rest stops where you can get up and move around. Don't try to drive too far in one day.

By Bus

Bus line policies about traveling with oxygen vary. Check with the bus line in advance. Ask whether the company will let you bring a companion on the trip without the cost of a second ticket if you have a doctor's note saying you need one.

By Train

Contact the railroad in advance to check what equipment you can bring, how much oxygen you will need, and whether you will need a traveling companion. Have an alternate power source and do not rely solely on the train's available electrical power. Be sure to get a seat in the non-smoking section.

Cruise Ships

Check with the cruise line about its policy on supplemental oxygen—some ships may provide it. If not, you will need to give your oxygen supplier plenty of notice to supply enough oxygen for the whole trip or arrange for refills at ports of call. Ask your supply company if it can provide you with an oxygen-conserving device for longer trips. Some companies, such as Medical Travel, Inc., organize cruises especially for people with lung disease (visit online at: www.MedicalTravel.org). ■

Compressed gas. Gas oxygen is stored under pressure in steel or aluminum canisters and must be purchased from a supplier. Larger canisters are usually used in the home; smaller ones are used when away from home. Normally, the outflow of oxygen from the canister is constant, but some systems have an oxygen-conserving device that releases oxygen only when you inhale. When using portable canisters, learn how long each one will last so you can time your outings accordingly.

Liquid oxygen. Liquid oxygen is stored at a very cold temperature; it returns to its gaseous state when released from the container. Like compressed gas, liquid oxygen must be purchased and stored in canisters and may include an oxygen-conserving device. Liquid oxygen is more portable than compressed gas because larger amounts can be stored in smaller containers. It is therefore often preferred by more active people. However, it has a limited shelf life and is more expensive than compressed gas.

Oxygen concentrators. An electric device called an oxygen concentrator can be used to extract oxygen from room air, which is about 20% oxygen. Oxygen concentrators are easier to maintain than other forms of oxygen therapy, and they may be ideal for people who spend most of their time at home. However, they are not suitable for everyone. They are not portable, some of them emit heat and are noisy, and the concentration of oxygen is lower than that in purchased gas or liquid oxygen. In addition, a backup source of oxygen is necessary in case of power failure.

The delivery method. In most cases, oxygen is delivered to the nose via a cannula—a 2-pronged tube device that connects to the oxygen canister or concentrator and rests just inside the nostrils. The tubing can either rest on the ears or be attached to eyeglasses. Some people purchase eyeglass frames with a built-in cannula to make oxygen therapy a little less apparent. Cannulas allow a person to eat and drink while still receiving oxygen. A mask, which fits over the nose and mouth, may be better suited for someone who needs a high flow of oxygen. Also, some people who normally use a nasal cannula find a mask more effective when they have nasal congestion or irritation caused by a cold.

Some people may choose to receive oxygen directly into the lungs through a catheter inserted into a surgically created hole in the trachea (windpipe). The procedure is most appropriate for people who require a high flow of oxygen because these individuals often use less oxygen when it is delivered directly into the lungs. The catheter needs meticulous daily cleaning, however, so that mucus does not collect on the tip of the device and block the trachea.

Using oxygen comfortably. Most people adjust very well to using oxygen, although a few adjustments may be necessary to increase comfort. Oxygen can be very drying to the body, especially to the nose. There are several ways to relieve this dryness. First, distilled water is often added to the oxygen to increase moisture, especially at higher flow rates. To treat a dry nose, you can apply an over-the-counter water-based lubricant (the pharmacist can give you a product recommendation) to the nose several times a day. Also, try to inhale through the nose, rather than the mouth, which wastes oxygen and can cause dry mouth. Alternatively, to relieve a sore or uncomfortable nose, try putting the cannula in your mouth for 2–3 hours several times a day to give your nose a rest.

Using oxygen effectively. Oxygen can be dangerous if not used and monitored carefully. It is flammable, so no one should smoke while someone is using oxygen nearby. Stay at least 5 feet away from open flames such as gas stoves, lighted fireplaces, and candles. Also, avoid flammable products such as aerosol sprays, paint thinners, and rubbing alcohol. Vapor rubs and petroleum jelly are also flammable and should be kept away from the oxygen canisters. Keep a fire extinguisher nearby, and let your local fire department know that oxygen is being used in the house.

When beginning home oxygen therapy, ask a representative from the medical supply company to come to your home and show you (and family members) how to use the equipment properly. Ask for specific instructions on how to clean and maintain the equipment. Finally, make sure you always have access to the oxygen. Order the next supply early enough to ensure that it arrives before you need it. Keep your medical supply company's emergency phone numbers accessible in case of an equipment failure. And alert your electric company that you have electrical oxygen equipment in your home—you should receive priority service in the event of a power failure. If traveling, make arrangements to have oxygen available on airline flights and in your destination city or country. For more information on traveling with oxygen, see the feature on page 28.

When to call your doctor. If you are on oxygen and develop confusion, headaches, or drowsiness, you may be getting too much oxygen and need to have your carbon dioxide levels checked. Blue fingernails or lips indicate low blood oxygen levels. Any of these symptoms should prompt an immediate call to your doctor.

Lung volume reduction surgery. Some people with emphysema may benefit from surgery called lung volume reduction surgery to remove diseased lung tissue. The procedure is believed to create more space in the chest cavity for the working lung tissue to expand. The procedure appears to prolong life in people with emphysema that predominantly affects the upper lobes and reduces exercise capacity. Medicare started covering the procedure for this group of people in 2003.

Lung transplantation. Another option for people with emphysema is lung transplantation. More than 1,000 lung transplants are performed annually in the United States. About 60% of these procedures involve a single lung (unilateral), while 40% involve both lungs (bilateral). Unilateral transplants are reserved for people with emphysema or pulmonary fibrosis (chronic inflammation and progressive scarring of the walls of the air sacs); bilateral transplants are used primarily in those with cystic fibrosis (an

NEW RESEARCH

Female Lung Transplant Recipients at Greater Risk of Acute Lung Injury

Female lung transplant recipients are significantly more likely to suffer from a type of injury to the transplanted lung called primary graft dysfunction than male lung transplant patients, according to a new study. Primary graft dysfunction is an acute severe lung injury that occurs within the first 72 hours after a transplant.

The study found that female lung transplant recipients who received a lung from either a male or female donor were almost 60% more likely to suffer from primary graft dysfunction, compared with male recipients who received their lung from a male donor.

The study included data on all 7,482 adult lung transplants performed in the U.S. from 1994–2002. The researchers took into account factors such as the donor's age, race, and cause of death, and the recipient's age, race, and reason for lung transplant, as well as the size-matching between the donor and recipient.

Overall, approximately 10% of transplant recipients suffered from primary graft dysfunction, which is associated with a high death rate, prolonged hospital stay, and other serious complications.

Still needed is further investigation into why the risk of primary graft dysfunction is increased in women.

AMERICAN THORACIC SOCIETY INTERNATIONAL CONFERENCE
Abstract 4691
May 2005

inherited disease in infants, children, and young adults that causes the body to produce an abnormally thick, sticky mucus which clogs the lungs and leads to life-threatening lung infections), patients with bronchiectasis, or select emphysema patients.

The scarcity of donor lungs and the risks of the procedure necessitate extensive evaluation of potential candidates for lung transplantation. Candidates must meet disease-specific criteria for severe (end-stage) lung disease and yet be able to survive the wait for one or both donor lungs and the rigors of the operation and post-operative period.

In 1998, international guidelines established an upper age limit of 64 years for unilateral transplants and 59 for bilateral transplants. Transplants cannot be performed in people with major disease in other organs, including HIV infection, cancer (other than basal or squamous cell skin cancers) diagnosed within the past 2 years, positive tests for hepatitis B antigen, or hepatitis C infection with liver disease. Lung transplantation may not be suitable for people who are obese or have severe osteoporosis.

Lung transplant patients are required to take medications for the rest of their life to suppress the immune system and prevent it from rejecting the transplanted lung(s). After successful transplantation, patients may experience some limitations in exercise tolerance but usually not enough to interfere with normal daily activities or adversely affect quality of life. The 5-year survival rate following lung transplantation is approximately 50%. The survival rate is highest in those treated for underlying emphysema and lowest in those treated for idiopathic pulmonary fibrosis (progressive scarring of the lungs in which the cause is unknown) or pulmonary hypertension. The most common cause of rejection, and the most dangerous complication of transplantation, is a condition called bronchiolitis obliterans, in which the bronchioles become blocked. Other common complications are infections and adverse effects of the immunosuppressive drugs.

SLEEP APNEA

Sleep apnea is a disorder characterized by repeated episodes of breathing cessation (apnea) during sleep. These episodes last from 10 seconds to nearly a minute and occur throughout the night. Periods of apnea end with a brief partial arousal that can disrupt sleep hundreds of times a night.

A 2003 study in the *Journal of the American Medical Association*

NEW RESEARCH

Death From Sleep Apnea More Common During Sleep

People with obstructive sleep apnea have a significantly increased risk of sudden death from heart problems during sleep, new research suggests. This contrasts with the dip in sudden death from heart problems during sleep in people who do not have sleep apnea and in the general population.

Researchers reviewed the records of 112 sleep study participants who had subsequently died suddenly from cardiac causes. The researchers compared the rates of sudden death during various times of day from cardiac causes among people with sleep apnea with rates of sudden death among people without sleep apnea, rates in the general population, and expectations according to chance.

In more than half of those participants with sleep apnea, sudden death from cardiac causes occurred between 10 p.m. and 6 a.m. By contrast, the people without sleep apnea had a day-night pattern of sudden death from cardiac causes very similar to that in the general population, with a peak in sudden death from cardiac causes from 6 a.m. to noon.

The risk of sudden death from cardiac causes during sleep hours was 40% higher overall in people with severe apnea, compared to people with mild-to-moderate sleep apnea.

THE NEW ENGLAND JOURNAL OF MEDICINE
Volume 352, page 1206
March 24, 2005

suggests that sleep apnea affects about 7% of the population. Indeed, an estimated 18 million Americans have obstructive sleep apnea, yet 95% of them are undiagnosed and untreated. Sleep apnea is about twice as common in men as in women.

Causes

Sleep apnea results from either a collapse and blockage of the upper airway during sleep, or a central nervous system abnormality that interferes with the drive to breathe. Some people have an anatomical abnormality that narrows the upper airway, such as large tonsils, excess fat in the tissues around the throat, or an enlarged tongue. A large neck or collar size (more than 17 inches in men or 16 inches in women) is strongly linked to sleep apnea. Obesity, older age, weakness of the airway muscles, hypothyroidism (insufficient production of thyroid hormone), and cigarette smoking are additional risk factors. Consuming alcohol or sedatives before sleeping can further reduce the activity of the airway muscles.

Symptoms

The most pervasive and troublesome symptom of sleep apnea is excessive daytime sleepiness caused by poor sleep. People with sleep apnea may fall asleep during the day while reading or even while driving, so there is a major risk of motor vehicle accidents. They may also suffer from memory loss and personality changes. Although loud snoring is a common sign of sleep apnea, snoring itself does not indicate obstructive sleep apnea.

More than half of those with sleep apnea also have high blood pressure, and their blood pressure does not fall during sleep as it does in most people. Sleep apnea has been shown to be an independent, treatable cause of high blood pressure.

The heart rate tends to slow dramatically during periods of apnea, then rise rapidly when breathing resumes. Some evidence suggests that periods of apnea and the resulting low levels of oxygen in the blood, along with persistently high blood pressure, increase the risk of coronary heart disease. Researchers are currently studying this link.

Diagnosis

Obtaining a sleep history is key to recognizing sleep apnea. Input from a person's bed partner can be especially important, because the partner is likely to notice snoring associated with frequent periods of apnea. A definitive diagnosis usually requires the

NEW RESEARCH

Men with Severe Sleep Apnea Have Higher Risk of Heart Problems

Men with untreated severe obstructive sleep apnea have a higher incidence of fatal and non-fatal heart problems compared to other men. But, according to a new study, the risk of heart problems is reduced when apnea is treated with continuous positive airway pressure (CPAP), the common therapy for the condition.

The study included 264 healthy men, 377 men who snored but did not have sleep apnea, 403 with untreated mild to moderate sleep apnea, 235 with untreated severe sleep apnea, and 372 with sleep apnea who were treated with CPAP. Participants were followed up at least once a year for an average of 10 years.

The researchers found that men with untreated severe sleep apnea were almost 3 times as likely as healthy participants to suffer from a fatal heart attack or stroke, and more than 3 times as likely to have a non-fatal heart attack or stroke or to require heart surgery.

Men with sleep apnea who were treated with CPAP had about one-third the risk of having a fatal heart problem compared to men with untreated severe sleep apnea.

THE LANCET
Volume 365, page 1046
March 19, 2005

Ordering Drugs From Canada?

Be safe!

If you are taking medication for lung disease, there's a good chance that you also are taking drugs for other conditions—and that means you're spending a lot on prescriptions.

"How to buy less expensive medications is one of the top questions I get from my patients," says Johns Hopkins lung specialist Peter B. Terry, M.D., author of this White Paper.

One way to purchase drugs at a reduced cost is to buy them online or by phone from Canadian pharmacies. The U.S. Food and Drug Administration (FDA) opposes foreign drug purchases, warning that these sales pose serious safety problems. While importing Canadian drugs is against U.S. policy, the FDA has said that it will not prosecute individuals who import small amounts (3 months or less) for personal use. However, several major drug manufacturers have stopped supplies to Canadian wholesalers who sell their products to pharmacies that sell to Americans, making it more difficult to obtain some popular medications.

This opposition has not stopped some states from launching websites to help their residents buy less expensive prescription drugs from Canada. One such site is www.I-SaveRx.net, designed to help residents of Illinois, Wisconsin, Missouri, Kansas, and Vermont buy less expensive drugs from Canada, Britain, and Ireland. Other states with similar websites include Minnesota, New Hampshire, and North Dakota. There are also plenty of other online Canadian pharmacies that residents of any state can order from.

If you are considering ordering drugs from Canada, remember that the FDA cannot guarantee the safety of those medicines.

The FDA's concerns include:

- **Quality assurance.** Medicines that have not been approved for sale in the United States may not have been manufactured under quality assurance procedures designed to produce a safe and effective product.
- **Counterfeit potential.** Some imported medicines—even those that have the name of a product approved in the United States—may, in fact, be counterfeit versions that are unsafe or ineffective.
- **Presence of untested substances.** Some imported medicines and their ingredients, although legal in foreign countries, may not have been evaluated for safety and effectiveness in the United States. These products may be addictive or contain other dangerous substances.
- **Risks of unsupervised use.** Some medicines, whether imported or not, are unsafe when taken without adequate medical supervision. You may need a medical evaluation to ensure that the medicine is appropriate for you and your condition. Or you may require medical checkups to make sure that you are taking the medicine properly, to assess whether it is working for you, and to check for unexpected or life-threatening side effects.
- **Labeling and language issues.** The medicine's label, including instructions for use and possible side effects, may be in a language you do not understand and may make medical claims or suggest specific uses that have not been adequately evaluated for safety and effectiveness.
- **Lack of information.** An imported medicine may not have information that would allow you to be treated promptly and correctly for a dangerous side effect caused by the medicine.

The American Association for Retired Persons (AARP), the leading non-profit, non-partisan membership organization for people aged 50 years and over in the United States, does not encourage Americans to

patient to spend a night in a hospital sleep laboratory to undergo sleep studies (polysomnography). Polysomnography involves monitoring brain waves to determine which stages of sleep are associated with episodes of apnea, as well as observing heart rhythms, airflow and breathing patterns, eye and leg movements, and blood oxygen levels. In some people, a pulse oximeter to record blood oxygen levels while sleeping at home can replace expensive sleep lab studies. A pulse oximeter test that shows low blood oxygen levels during sleep can aid in the diagnosis of sleep apnea, but a normal result does not rule out the possibility of the disorder.

break the present drug importation law. But with an estimated 2 million Americans already buying prescription drugs from Canada, the organization has come up with guidelines to help consumers minimize their risk and ensure that the drugs they receive are the ones their doctors have prescribed.

If after considering the risks, you decide to proceed with ordering drugs from a Canadian pharmacy, AARP recommends that you pick a pharmacy that:

• **Provides its license number on its website** and the name of the Canadian regulatory agency that granted the license so that you can check the pharmacy's authenticity.

• **Displays the seals of the Canadian International Pharmacy Association (CIPA**; see www.ciparx.ca/) **or Internet and Mail-Order Pharmacy Accreditation Commission (IMPAC**; see www.impacsurvey.org/). These organizations set standards for safety and service among Canadian mail-order pharmacies that sell to Americans. Those that meet the standards receive accreditation.

• **Requires a prescription from your doctor.** Reputable pharmacies may allow you to fax in a prescription but will then either confirm the prescription by a phone call to your doctor's office or wait until they receive the original one in the mail before filling your order.

• **Requires you to submit details of your medical history** and clearly states the pharmacy's policies for ensuring medical and personal privacy.

• **Requires you to have taken a drug for at least 1 month** before you order by mail so that you and your doctor know the medication is working and is safe for you.

• **Provides a full mailing address and a toll-free phone number** on its website so that you can call a pharmacist to ask any questions you may have.

• **Explains differences between American and Canadian drug names and labeling** and why the pharmacy does not sell some drugs.

• **Normally sends drugs in the manufacturer's original container, with seals intact.** An exception to this rule occurs when the quantity of pills in the manufacturer's own container exceeds a 90-day supply. In these cases, drugs may arrive in ordinary pharmacy bottles.

• **Sends drugs with labeling** that includes strength, dosing directions, expiration date, appropriate warnings, and a Drug Identification Number (DIN) that shows the drug has been approved by the Canadian government health authorities.

• **Displays on its website full information about shipping fees, payment policies, and refunds.** Reputable pharmacies offer secure (encrypted) online payment for credit cards, alternative options for payment (such as electronic fund transfers and regular checks), and do not charge any separate fees except for shipping.

• **Charges the cost of the drugs to your credit card only when the drugs are shipped**, not when the order is first placed.

• **Refunds your money or reships drugs immediately** if your order does not arrive.

If you're wondering where to start looking for pharmacies online, visit www.pharmacychecker.com, a website run by an independent American consumer research group that provides ratings and price comparisons for more than 40 online pharmacies based mainly in the United States and Canada. This site rates them on a scale of 1–5 and notes whether a pharmacy is licensed, requires a prescription, provides its address and phone number, and offers personal privacy and payment security. The site compares prices for more than 1,000 drugs at these pharmacies and gives details on shipping fees and delivery times. ■

Treatment

Lifestyle measures that may reduce sleep apnea include losing weight (for overweight and obese people), avoiding alcohol and sedatives at bedtime, quitting smoking, and sleeping on your side or in a more upright position. If hypothyroidism is present, treating it may help reduce the apnea.

If these measures are unsuccessful, continuous positive airway pressure (CPAP) may be necessary. This technique, which involves wearing a nasal mask that delivers a steady stream of air to maintain airway pressure and keep the airways open, is effective in 80–90% of people. However, the mask is cumbersome and can cause nasal dryness, nasal congestion, and skin irritation. Use of a humidifier or a properly fitting mask can alleviate some of these problems.

Some people benefit from a dental appliance that helps maintain an open airway by keeping the jaw and tongue in a forward position while sleeping. In addition, carefully selected people who cannot tolerate CPAP may benefit from uvulopalatopharyngoplasty, a surgical procedure that increases the size of the upper airway by removing the uvula (the tag-like structure that hangs down from the back of the throat) and any excessive tissue surrounding it. This procedure is successful in only 40–50% of people, typically those with mild cases of sleep apnea. Tonsillectomy, surgical treatment of other upper airway obstructions, and facial reconstructive procedures are helpful in some cases. In addition, a 2002 study revealed that boosting the heart rate during sleep can reduce sleep apnea; this may prove to be a practical treatment for people with pacemakers.

Finally, in 2004 the U.S. Food and Drug Administration (FDA) approved a drug called modafanil (Provigil) to help people with sleep apnea and other sleep disorders stay awake. Modafanil was originally approved in 1998 to treat narcolepsy. The most common side effects are headache, nausea, nervousness, stuffy nose, diarrhea, back pain, anxiety, trouble sleeping at night, dizziness, and upset stomach.

INTERSTITIAL LUNG DISEASE

Interstitial lung disease (ILD) refers to a group of more than 200 chronic disorders in which lung tissue is damaged, the walls of the air sacs become inflamed, and scarring (fibrosis) begins in the interstitium—the tissue between the air sacs. Though many of the disorders are uncommon, taken together ILD is a frequent cause of respiratory problems, accounting for 15% of all lung disorders evaluated by pulmonologists.

The lung scarring associated with ILD leads to stiffness that makes breathing difficult and interferes with the transfer of oxygen in the lungs. The pace of lung deterioration varies greatly from person to person. Interstitial lung disease includes disorders such as pulmonary sarcoidosis, bronchiolitis obliterans organizing pneumonia, asbestosis, and silicosis. Pulmonary sarcoidosis is an inflammatory disease in which granulomas—small clusters of cells—develop in the lungs and adjacent lymph nodes (small, round-shaped groups of immune defense cells that help prevent the spread of infection and protect the bloodstream from viral and bacterial invasion). Pulmonary sarcoidosis can increase lung stiffness, which reduces lung volumes. Bronchiolitis obliterans organizing pneumonia refers to inflammation with blockage of the bronchioles (the small airways in the lungs that branch from the large ones). Asbestosis and silicosis refer to damage caused by exposure to dust from asbestos and silica, respectively. Idiopathic pulmonary fibrosis is a condition of unknown (idiopathic) cause in which progressive scarring of the lungs markedly compromises day-to-day function.

Causes

A variety of factors can injure the air sacs and result in ILD. Possible causes include:

- Certain prescription drugs (including chemotherapy drugs and cardiovascular medications)
- Exposure to environmental toxins
- Infectious agents (such as viruses, bacteria, or fungi)
- Substances that trigger allergic or hypersensitivity reactions (such as certain proteins found in bird droppings) in susceptible persons
- Connective tissue diseases, such as scleroderma, rheumatoid arthritis, and lupus, all of which can cause inflammation and scarring of organs, including the lungs
- The spread of cancer to the lungs from other parts of the body.

In many cases, the cause of lung injury is unknown.

Symptoms

Symptoms vary widely depending on the specific disease, but most people with ILD become short of breath when they exert themselves and have a persistent cough that does not produce phlegm. Fatigue, loss of appetite, and weight loss are common in many types of ILD; wheezing, chest pain, coughing up blood, and fever are also possible. The disease may only last for several weeks, but, more commonly, symptoms persist for months or years.

Diagnosis

Abnormalities on a chest x-ray may be the first evidence of ILD, but the irregularities are often not specific to a particular disorder. For

NEW RESEARCH

Treating Sleep Apnea Lowers Glucose Levels in People With Diabetes

People with type 2 diabetes who also have obstructive sleep apnea can lower their glucose levels by using the treatment known as continuous positive airway pressure, or CPAP, according to a new study. Snoring and sleep apnea have been associated with the development of diabetes in several studies.

Researchers studied 25 people with type 2 diabetes who were referred for sleep apnea treatment. Their glucose levels were measured before and after CPAP therapy. When they received at least 4 hours of CPAP treatment daily, their glucose levels went down.

Because of the high prevalence of obesity and sleep disordered breathing in diabetic patients, these results emphasize the benefits of treating sleep apnea. They also suggest that treating severe sleep apnea in people with early signs of diabetes (impaired glucose tolerance or impaired fasting glucose levels) might prevent or delay progression to full-blown diabetes.

ARCHIVES OF INTERNAL MEDICINE
Volume 165, page 447
February 28, 2005

What is a Bronchoscopy?

A closer look at the lungs

The bronchoscopy is an examination that allows your doctor to see the airways of your lungs and take samples of mucus or tissue from your lungs. A thin, tube-like instrument, called a bronchoscope, is put through your nose or mouth and down into your lung's air passages. The tube has a mini-camera at its tip that transmits pictures back to a video screen or camera. The instrument also has a passageway that lets the doctor remove mucus and cell samples from the lining of the lung and collect a small sample of tissue with a mini-cutting device.

Your doctor may order a bronchoscopy for one of the following reasons:

- To follow up on an abnormal chest x-ray
- To find the cause of certain infections such as tuberculosis, AIDS-related pneumonias, or pneumonia following organ transplantation
- To investigate and remove a blockage in the airways
- To find out the cause of bleeding in the lung.

What Are the Risks of Bronchoscopy?

Bronchoscopy is a safe test, and serious complications are rare. Minor complications that can occur include discomfort while the bronchoscope is being passed through your nose, throat, and air passages, and a tickling feeling that may cause you to cough. To reduce this discomfort, the doctor will spray a local anesthetic in your nose or throat to numb the area. Sedatives given before the procedure also reduce discomfort.

Although bronchoscopy is safe, in rare cases the airways can be injured by the bronchoscope (especially if the lung is already very inflamed or diseased) or a lung puncture can occur, causing an air leak around the lung (called a pneumothorax), which can lead to lung collapse. The bronchoscope can also injure a tumor in the airways.

Another complication is bleeding after a biopsy. Usually it is minor and will stop without treatment, but if needed, medication can be given through the instrument to stop the bleeding.

How Do I Prepare for a Bronchoscopy?

Your stomach needs to be empty before the bronchoscopy to lessen certain risks, such as vomiting during the procedure. You will be told not to eat or drink anything (not even water) for 6 hours before the procedure. If you are taking any type of medication, ask your doctor whether you need to stop taking it beforehand. (If your doctor says it's okay to take your regular medications, you may drink a little water in order to take them.) If you have diabetes, your doctor may need to adjust your medication or insulin dose both before and after the procedure.

Before the bronchoscopy begins, you will be given a small amount of sedative intravenously in your hand or arm. As noted above, you will receive a local anesthetic for your nose and/or throat to help prevent coughing and gagging. If needed, you may receive additional sedation through the needle in your vein. You will also be connected to a heart and blood pressure monitor to check your vital signs during the procedure.

What Happens During the Procedure?

You will probably be lying down during the procedure. The doctor will slowly put the bronchoscope through your mouth and throat, through your vocal cords to your windpipe, and down into your lungs.

Any urge to cough or feelings of discomfort should be temporary. Your doctor will stop and let you catch your breath before continuing. Take slow, shallow breaths through your mouth,

example, pulmonary function tests typically show a decrease in total lung capacity—the amount of air in the lungs after a deep inhalation. Another common abnormality is a decrease in diffusion capacity—a measurement of how well gas passes across the membranes in the lungs. Again, these deviations do not distinguish among the various underlying causes of ILD.

The results of high-resolution chest CT scans may be helpful in people suspected of having ILD. For example, a scan showing changes in which the severely damaged lung resembles a honeycomb on the edge may eliminate the need for a lung biopsy because it is so specific for one form of ILD. In some cases, a specific and do not talk (this will help prevent a sore throat). If needed, you will receive medication through the instrument to help relieve coughing.

The procedure can take anywhere from 15 minutes to 1 hour, depending on how long it takes for the medicine to kick in and what procedures the doctor needs to do.

What is the Recovery Time?
Recovery times vary from patient to patient. You will be observed until you are alert enough to leave. It is recommended that you bring someone along to drive you home.

You must wait 30 minutes to 1 hour before drinking anything, until the numbness wears off. It is unlikely that you will have any problems after the procedure; however, if you feel chest pain or increased shortness of breath, or cough up large amounts of blood once you leave the hospital, call your doctor right away. It is normal to cough up a small amount of blood for 1–2 days after the procedure.

When Do I Get the Results?
Your doctor can tell you how your airways look right away. You may get lab results within 1–4 days, but other results can take longer, depending on what was done during the bronchoscopy. ■

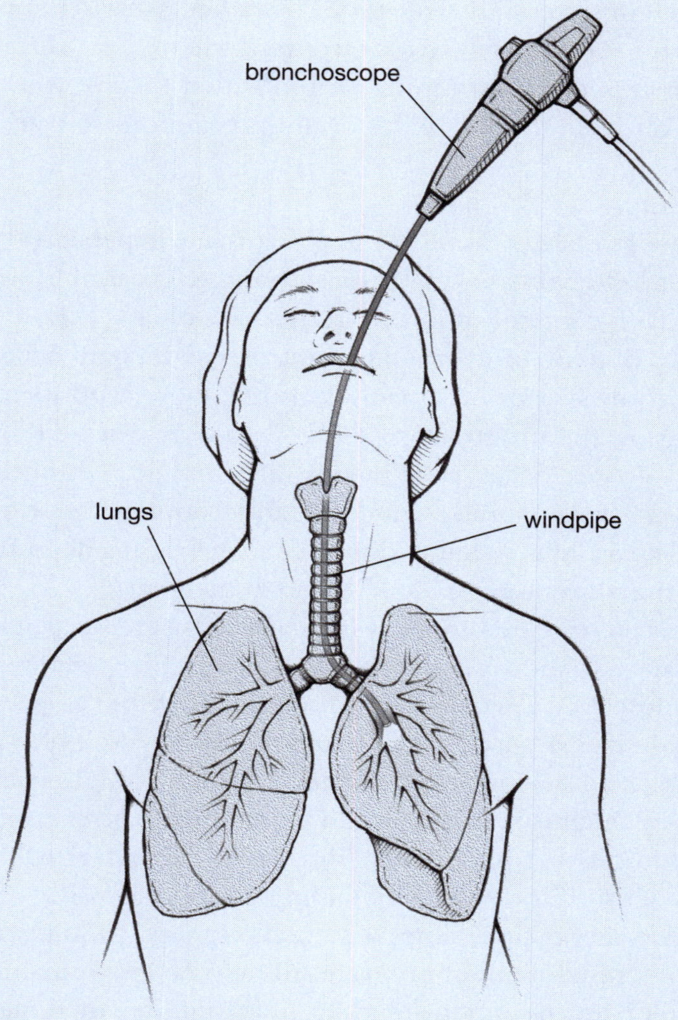

Bronchoscopy

diagnosis can be made from the examination of lung fluids obtained using bronchoalveolar lavage (washing out the lungs with a saline solution) during bronchoscopy—a procedure in which a thin, hollow, flexible tube is passed through the mouth and into the windpipe to allow viewing of the main airway passages.

In some cases, a lung biopsy may be necessary to make a definitive diagnosis and determine the severity of the disease. Least invasive is a biopsy done through a bronchoscope. This procedure can be done on an outpatient basis, but the small size of the tissue sample may not be sufficient for diagnosis. If this approach is inconclusive, an open surgical biopsy in a hospital would be necessary.

Prevention

Avoidance of potential triggers of ILD is key. Wearing appropriate masks and monitoring exposure to irritants in certain work environments (such as mining and jobs that involve working with asbestos or metal dusts) are important precautions to take.

Treatment

Several types of ILD, notably sarcoidosis and hypersensitivity reactions, get better on their own or respond to treatment with corticosteroids. Treatment of infections responsible for ILD, along with avoidance of toxin or allergen exposures, can be beneficial.

Unfortunately, for other causes of ILD, there is no specific treatment to slow the progression of the disease or reverse the damage that has already occurred. Further inflammation and scarring of lung tissue weaken lung function and can lead to right heart failure—heart failure that mainly affects the right side of the heart, slowing the movement of blood through the heart.

Corticosteroid treatment, which can be beneficial in treating pulmonary sarcoidosis, may be prescribed for people suffering from symptoms caused by other forms of ILD, but it is frequently unsuccessful. Chemotherapy drugs such as cyclophosphamide (Cytoxan, Neosar) or azathioprine (Imuran), anti-fibrotic agents such as colchicine, and interferon gamma have been tried in people with idiopathic pulmonary fibrosis, but an effective treatment remains elusive for this debilitating and progressive condition. Supportive care includes supplemental oxygen, adequate nutrition, pulmonary rehabilitation programs to help people remain as active as possible, and treatment of right heart failure. In some cases, a single or double lung transplant can be performed.

LUNG CANCER

Lung cancer was rare before the beginning of the 20th century, but it is now the most common cause of death from cancer among both men and women in the United States. An estimated 160,440 Americans died of lung cancer in 2004. Death rates are so high because lung cancer is difficult to treat and usually is not detected until it has already spread. Most cases occur in people between the ages of 45 and 75 who have been exposed to cigarette smoke or other pollutants for many years. Tragically, only about 15% of people with lung cancer are alive 5 years after diagnosis.

Lung cancer may be primary or secondary. Primary lung cancer, which originates in the lungs, is grouped into two broad categories: small cell carcinoma (about 20% of cases) and non-small cell carcinoma (about 80%). Because small cell carcinoma spreads especially quickly and is more difficult to treat, most people with this type die within a year of diagnosis. Primary lung cancer can spread to nearly any organ.

Cancer may also spread to the lungs from other sites in the body, called secondary lung cancer. These types of tumors are usually incurable, in which case palliative treatments are used. Palliative care is aimed at delaying the progression of disease, relieving pain, and limiting disease complications, rather than curing the disease.

Causes

Smoking causes an estimated 87–90% of lung cancer cases. Smokers who quit (even after smoking for years) greatly reduce their risk (see "Quitting Smoking: Instant Benefits" on page 43). However, the risk remains, as the public was reminded of in August 2005 when former smoker Peter Jennings, ABC's news anchor, died of lung cancer. One recent study provided some of the first direct evidence of how cigarette smoking leads to lung cancer. Researchers found that the body converts a substance in cigarette smoke, called benzo[a]pyrene diol epoxide (BPDE), into a potent carcinogen.

Nonsmokers have only a small risk of developing lung cancer. One well-known nonsmoker recently diagnosed with lung cancer is Dana Reeve, widow of actor Christopher Reeve, who announced she had the disease in August 2005.

Several comprehensive reports have also concluded that passive smoking—inhaling the smoke from cigarettes smoked by others—can cause lung cancer in non-smokers. The presence of carcinogens in the smoke coming from the end of a burning cigarette (sidestream smoke), the presence of cigarette smoke particles in the homes of smokers, detection of tobacco-smoke components in the body fluids of nonsmokers, and the 30% increased incidence of lung cancer in the non-smoking spouses of smokers all support this conclusion. Some data suggest that passive smoking is one of the leading causes of preventable deaths in this country, if projected deaths from lung cancer and cardiovascular disease are counted together.

Exposure to toxic substances such as radon and asbestos can also lead to lung cancer. In fact, radon is estimated to be the leading cause of lung cancer among nonsmokers and the second leading cause overall.

NEW RESEARCH

Lung Cancer May Not Be Such a "Silent' Disease

Although lung cancer is often thought to be a "silent disease," with no symptoms appearing until it's too late for treatment, a new study finds that some lung cancer patients had symptoms for many months before they were diagnosed.

This study of 22 men and women recently diagnosed with lung cancer found that patients recalled having new symptoms for many months, typically during the year before their diagnosis, no matter what the stage of their disease when diagnosed.

Chest symptoms (cough, breathing changes, and chest pain) were common, as were feelings of fatigue/lethargy, weight loss, and eating changes. Most symptoms were not interpreted as serious by patients at the time, and were therefore not acted on. The patients' beliefs about health changes that could indicate lung cancer played a part in the delay in diagnosis.

Better insight into patients' perspectives on their experience before being diagnosed with lung cancer may help doctors to recognize patients with lung cancer earlier and more easily so that they can refer them for diagnosis and treatment as soon as possible.

THORAX
Volume 60, page 314
April 2005

Radon is a colorless, odorless gas formed naturally during the decay of uranium found in rocks and soil. Radon in the soil can pollute the air of a home by entering through cracks or other openings, usually in the basement. The incidence of lung cancer caused by radon is highest among miners, who are often exposed to high levels.

Asbestos is a fibrous mineral that was used in building materials until the 1980s. Chronic exposure to asbestos can cause both lung cancer and mesothelioma—a cancer involving the pleura (the membranes that cover the lungs). The combination of asbestos exposure and cigarette smoking is especially dangerous.

Air pollution, including traffic fumes and smokestack emissions, also may contribute to lung cancer.

Symptoms

Lung cancer produces such quiet symptoms in its early stages that it is typically diagnosed at an advanced stage. (For more information on possible early symptoms, see the "New Research" column on page 41.) Later in the disease, people often notice fatigue, poor appetite, and unexplained weight loss. These symptoms are common to many forms of cancer.

Symptoms specific to the growth and spread of lung cancer may include coughing up red or rust-colored phlegm, wheezing, and shortness of breath. Sometimes an infection in the lung behind the tumor that is obstructing the airway produces a fever. Invasion of cancerous cells into the pleura or other nearby structures can produce pain in the chest, shoulders, or arms. If the cancer spreads to surrounding tissues, it can lead to enlarged lymph nodes in the chest or neck and impingement of various nerves, resulting in hoarseness. Due to narrowing of the esophagus, a person may have difficulty swallowing. There may be swelling of the neck and face from blockage of blood flow from these areas to the heart. In about 30% of patients, lung cancer also causes clubbing of the fingers (a thickening of the fingertips and increased curvature of the fingernails).

Lung cancer often spreads to the liver and bone marrow, where it can interfere with the formation of blood cells. When it spreads to the bones, it causes pain and fractures, and when it spreads to the brain, it produces neurological symptoms such as seizures. Some lung cancer patients with small cell tumors may develop Cushing's syndrome, which produces such complications as osteoporosis, high blood pressure, and roundness of the face. Another

Quitting Smoking: Instant Benefits

Virtually the minute you quit smoking, your health begins to improve

The negative effects of smoking are clear: One in every 3 people who starts smoking will die prematurely of a smoking-related illness, according to the American Lung Association. And 1 in every 5 deaths stems directly from tobacco exposure. But the good news is that it's never too late to quit smoking. The benefits of smoking cessation begin within a few minutes of your last cigarette and continue for life, even for people with lung disease.

The Risks of Smoking

Although smoking's link to lung cancer is well known, the habit is even more likely to cause a range of other illnesses. According to a 2003 survey published in *Morbidity and Mortality Weekly Report*, some 8.6 million Americans were living with a major smoking-related illness in 2000. The most common of these was chronic bronchitis (35% of cases), emphysema (24%), heart attacks (19%), non-lung cancer (12%), strokes (8%), and lung cancer (1%).

The true number of people affected by smoking is probably much higher than the researchers stated because this study depended on people to report whether a doctor had ever told them they had a certain condition. People tend to underreport their own illnesses. In addition, the researchers did not look at non-debilitating conditions, such as impotence and sinusitis, that are often caused by cigarette smoking.

The Benefits of Quitting

Regardless of how long you smoked, your health begins to improve shortly after your last cigarette. And the longer you are smoke free, the greater the benefits become. The chart below lists a timeline of these health improvements. ■

Time Since Last Cigarette	Health Benefits
20 minutes	Elevated blood pressure levels begin to drop, and the temperature in your extremities begins to return to normal.
8 hours	You achieve normal blood levels of carbon monoxide.
1 day	Your risk of a heart attack begins to decline.
2 weeks–3 months	Circulation improves, and lung function increases, decreasing the risk of lung infections.
1–9 months	Shortness of breath, sinus congestion, coughing, and fatigue improve. A few months of smoking cessation improves lung function about 5% in patients with chronic obstructive pulmonary disease (COPD), and the risk of death from COPD declines.
1 year	Your risk of having a heart attack is cut in half.
5 years	The risk of cancer in the oral cavity and esophagus is already half that of continuing smokers, and the risk continues to decline with continued cessation.
5–15 years	The risk of a stroke becomes similar to that of a lifelong nonsmoker.
10 years	Your risk of developing lung cancer is 30–50% lower than it would be had you continued to smoke, and the risk continues to decline with continued abstinence. Also, you've significantly decreased your risk of developing cancer of the bladder, cervix, esophagus, kidney, mouth, pancreas, and throat.
10–15 years	Your odds of dying of any cause are the same as those of someone who never smoked.
15 years	Your risk of having a heart attack is the same as a lifelong nonsmoker.

possible complication of lung cancer is hypercalcemia—excessive blood levels of calcium—which can cause fatigue, muscle weakness, confusion, drowsiness, and coma.

Diagnosis

About 10% of lung cancers are discovered in people with no symptoms, usually when a chest x-ray is performed for another reason. However, the majority of lung cancers are diagnosed after a doctor requests testing for cancer based on a patient's medical history and the results of a physical examination.

Doctors usually do not recommend general screening for lung cancer in at-risk individuals (for example, smokers and former smokers). A standard chest x-ray is not sensitive enough to locate small tumors, and studies have shown that 2 screening methods—regular chest x-rays and phlegm examinations—do not decrease the number of deaths from lung cancer.

A recently developed technology called low-radiation-dose spiral computed tomography (spiral CT) is currently being investigated as a screening tool for lung cancer. Spiral CT generates a series of cross-sectional images of the lungs used to create a three-dimensional image. The radiation exposure from a spiral CT scan is slightly higher than a regular chest x-ray. It costs about $300, compared with $150 for the less accurate chest x-ray and $2,000 for the time-consuming positron emission tomography (PET) and magnetic resonance imaging (MRI) scans.

Spiral CT provides clear images and can be performed in about 20 seconds. In addition, the majority of lung cancers detected by spiral CT appear to be in the earliest, most treatable stage. But there are disadvantages to the imaging test. Because spiral CT cannot distinguish between non-cancerous tumors, it has a high rate of false positives, in which non-cancerous nodules (small lumps of tissue) are flagged as being possibly cancerous. This leads to unnecessary and risky lung biopsies and can turn a painless and relatively inexpensive test into a painful and expensive one. An analysis performed at Johns Hopkins and published in the *Journal of the American Medical Association* in 2003 suggested that the procedure is not yet cost-effective and that the risks outweigh the benefits.

Yet other studies suggest that spiral CT screening for lung cancer may benefit some populations, particularly current and former smokers over age 60. In 1 study of 1,000 asymptomatic smokers and former smokers, the scan detected 23 early-stage cancers; standard chest x-rays missed 83% of them. Spiral CT outperformed chest x-rays on all fronts, uncovering 3 times as many suspicious nodules and 4 times as many cancerous tumors. Of the 27 cancerous tumors found by spiral CT scans in the study, 26 were successfully removed.

A multi-center study of spiral CT is under way to evaluate the rate of false-positive results and the test's impact on long-term lung cancer cure rates.

A biopsy of cancerous tissue is essential for an accurate diagnosis of lung cancer. It also guides treatment decisions. A biopsy sample can be obtained from the suspicious area using bronchoscopy, in which a thin, hollow, flexible tube is passed through the mouth and into the windpipe to allow viewing of the main bronchial passages (see feature on page 38). Tissue is obtained either directly from an airway or by passing a needle through an airway into adjacent tumor tissue. Alternatively, a CT-scan-guided needle biopsy through the chest wall may be used to obtain tissue from a suspicious growth within the lung. In people with suspected lung cancer, a positive result for cancer generally is reliable. A negative result does not necessarily exclude cancer, however, and further testing is often necessary. This testing may include an open lung biopsy or a mediastinoscopy, in which the structures behind the breastbone in the chest cavity are examined. Common sites of cancer spread, such as the lymph nodes, bone marrow, and pleura, are suitable areas for biopsy.

Staging is a system for determining how much cancer a patient has and how far it has spread. Decisions about how the cancer is to be treated are based on the staging system. Imaging procedures—for example, CT, MRI, and PET scans—are important components of this evaluation.

Prevention

The best ways to prevent lung cancer are to avoid smoking and limit exposure to certain pollutants.

Smoking. Cigarette smoking is unquestionably the single greatest controllable risk factor for lung cancer and the most common preventable cause of all premature deaths in the United States. Half of all smokers die prematurely of diseases related to smoking. While smoking cigars and pipes greatly increases the danger of cancers of the mouth, pharynx, larynx, and esophagus, the risk of lung cancer is not as high as with cigarette smoking because smoke from pipes and cigars is usually not inhaled as deeply or as frequently as cigarette smoke. The risk of lung cancer is greatest in those who start smoking at an early age and smoke the most cigarettes daily.

NEW RESEARCH

Intensive Smoking Cessation Programs Improve Long-Term Survival of Smokers

According to a study of 5,900 smokers, intensive smoking cessation programs can significantly improve long-term survival among smokers.

The study followed middle-aged smokers who had mild to moderately abnormal lung function but who were otherwise healthy. Participants were assigned to either a 10-week intensive smoking cessation program or to usual care (no intervention). The intervention program included behavior modification and nicotine gum, with a 5-year maintenance program to minimize relapse

After 5 years, 22% of participants in the smoking cessation program were still ex-smokers, with nearly 90% of this group still smoke-free after 11 years. In contrast, only about 5% of those who did not receive the intervention were still smoke-free after 5 years. After an average of 14.5 years, the death rate among those in the smoking cessation group was about 15% lower than the death rate of the no-intervention group.

The researchers also found that death rates of sustained quitters compared to smokers were nearly one-third lower for heart disease and less than half for lung cancer.

ANNALS OF INTERNAL MEDICINE
Volume 142, page 233
February 15, 2005

Because the risk of lung and other cancers gradually diminishes after smoking is discontinued, smokers can benefit from quitting at any age. The benefit of smoking cessation in reducing the risk of lung cancer becomes evident after about 5 years. The risk of developing lung cancer continues to decrease the longer a person does not smoke, but it does not fall all the way down to the level of someone who never smoked.

Radon. Many studies have examined the risk of lung cancer posed by radon in the home. Data from miners suggest that household levels of radon might account for about 15% of lung cancer deaths, an estimate supported by studies that have directly measured the risk of indoor radon. The U.S. Environmental Protection Agency (EPA) has recommended measuring radon levels in homes and reducing the levels when they exceed 4 picocuries per liter (pCi/L) over a year, a level estimated to be present in about 5% of American homes. Some critics have disagreed with this EPA recommendation, arguing that these levels of radon do not pose a significant risk and that attention should be focused on finding the homes with the highest levels. Recently, researchers estimated that reducing radon levels in all homes with readings higher than 4 pCi/L would result in 2–4% fewer lung cancer deaths.

To determine whether radon levels are high in your area, call your local EPA office. Taking a radon measurement in an individual house is the only way to definitively know the radon level, and several inexpensive kits are available in most hardware stores. Etched-track or electret detectors are good choices; the best of these kits take measurements over at least a 3-month period. The label on the kit should say that it meets EPA requirements or is certified by the state. If it is necessary to reduce radon levels in your home, contact a state-certified contractor or one who has passed the EPA Radon Contractor Proficiency Program.

Dietary measures. Since damage of DNA by free radicals is considered one of the causes of many types of cancer, it was hoped that antioxidant supplements or an increased intake of antioxidant-rich foods might reduce the risk of lung cancer. A Scandinavian study, however, found that beta-carotene supplements actually increased the risk of lung cancer in cigarette smokers. Currently, no dietary measures are known to diminish the risk of lung cancer.

Treatment

The 3 options for treating lung cancer—surgery, chemotherapy, and radiation therapy—may be used alone or in combination. The choice

NEW RESEARCH

Avastin Plus Chemotherapy Prolongs Survival in Advanced Lung Cancer

Patients with non-small cell lung cancer who took bevacizumab (Avastin) and had chemotherapy took longer to relapse than patients who received chemotherapy alone, according to a new study.

The study included 434 patients receiving combination therapy and 444 receiving chemotherapy alone. The average length of time before recurrence in patients receiving combination treatment was 6.4 months, compared with 4.5 months in the chemotherapy-only group. After one year of treatment, 51.9% of patients on combination treatment were alive, compared with 43.7% on chemotherapy alone. At 2 years, 22.1% of those on the combination were alive, compared with 16.9% on chemotherapy alone.

The most serious side effect was life-threatening or fatal bleeding, mainly from the lungs. This occurred in 1.7% of patients in the Avastin group but was nonexistent in the chemotherapy-only group.

The researchers concluded that adding Avastin to chemotherapy in people with non-small cell lung cancer provides a significant survival advantage and has tolerable toxicity. The trial did not include people with squamous cell lung cancer because an earlier Avastin trial that included patients with this type of lung cancer had shown life-threatening bleeding rates of up to 10%.

AMERICAN SOCIETY OF CLINICAL ONCOLOGY
Abstract LBA4
May 2005

of treatment depends on a number of factors, including the size and location of the tumor, whether the cancer is small cell or non-small cell, the physical condition of the patient, and whether the cancer has spread to lymph nodes or further. Because of the complexity of treatment, people with lung cancer should discuss their options with a multidisciplinary team of experts, which includes a pulmonologist, a thoracic surgeon, medical and radiation oncologists, and other health professionals (see feature on page 7).

Surgery. All people with lung cancer should be evaluated for possible surgery because surgery is the most effective treatment for non-small cell cancer. Resectability and operability are major considerations in deciding whether a person is a good candidate for surgery. A resectable tumor is one that can be removed in its entirety. If the tumor has spread extensively or is too close to vital structures, such as the heart or major blood vessels, it is no longer resectable. The decision that a tumor is not resectable is usually based on information from both the biopsy and scans. A tumor is considered operable if the patient is able to undergo the surgical procedure safely and can tolerate the extent of resection necessary for a cure. The patient's lung function and the presence of other diseases are key factors in determining operability.

Surgery may involve removal of a lobe or an entire lung. A hospital stay of 1–2 weeks is usually required. People with otherwise healthy lungs can often resume normal activities after a period of recuperation. Most people need 2–6 months to recover.

Chemotherapy. Chemotherapy is individualized for each patient and may involve administration of a combination of several drugs given in 4–6 cycles. The drug cisplatin (Platinol) used to be the standard treatment for non-small cell lung cancer. Now a second drug, such as gemcitabine (Gemzar), vinorelbine (Navelbine), paclitaxel (Taxol), or docetaxel (Taxotere) is added to boost cisplatin's effectiveness. Sometimes a less toxic drug called carboplatin (Paraplatin) is substituted for cisplatin. Like most chemotherapy regimens, these combinations usually cause temporary but severe side effects that may include nausea, vomiting, loss of appetite, hair loss, mouth sores, severe diarrhea, fatigue, and low resistance to infection. Other drug regimens for non-small cell lung cancer are currently being studied.

In May 2003, the FDA approved a new drug—gefitinib (Iressa)—for the treatment of patients with non-small cell lung cancer who had failed 2 or more courses of chemotherapy. In December 2004, however, the FDA announced that a large clinical trial comparing

NEW RESEARCH

Fit Elderly Patients Can Get Aggressive Treatment for Small Cell Lung Cancer

Survival rates among patients aged 70 and older with small cell lung cancer who are treated with radiation and chemotherapy are similar to younger patients who receive the same aggressive treatment, a new study finds.

The 263 study participants (54 of them 70 years or older) with limited-stage small cell lung cancer (LD-SCLC) received chemotherapy plus radiation once or twice a day. The researchers compared how long it took for tumors to start growing again, survival, and the severity of side effects among older vs. younger patients.

Age was not a factor in how quickly the tumors recurred. The differences in survival were slightly higher among the younger age group, but were not significant—2 years after treatment, 48% of younger patients and 33% of older patients were still alive. Five years after treatment, 22% of younger patients and 17% of older patients were still alive.

Patients in both age groups had similarly severe side effects, such as nausea, vomiting, irritation of the esophagus, and low white blood cell and platelet counts. Elderly patients had more cases of pneumonitis, a breathing problem that requires treatment with a ventilator or continuous oxygen.

CANCER
Volume 103, page 2348
April 25, 2005

Iressa with a placebo (a "dummy" pill) in patients with non-small cell lung cancer who had failed other courses of cancer therapy showed no survival benefit from taking Iressa.

Cisplatin plus etoposide (VePesid, Etopophos, Toposar) is usually considered the optimal chemotherapy regimen for small cell lung cancer, but researchers are studying many other possible approaches as well.

Radiation. External radiation may be the main form of treatment for people unable to tolerate surgery and for those whose cancer has spread beyond the reach of surgical removal. Radiation is administered 5 days a week for 4–8 weeks. It may be directed to areas of cancer in the lung that cannot be removed with surgery, or it may be used to treat cancer that has spread to the brain or bones or cancer that compresses the spinal cord. Side effects of external radiation include nausea and vomiting, local skin irritation, and fatigue.

Novel Approaches. Two innovative approaches being tested for lung cancer treatment are vaccination and gene therapy.

Vaccination. The GVAX lung cancer vaccine is made from a patient's own tumor cells. These cells are genetically modified to secrete a hormone that stimulates the immune system to attack the tumor. Two 75-person trials with the vaccine are currently under way.

Gene therapy. Researchers at the University of Texas M. D. Anderson Cancer Center and the University of Texas Southwestern Medical Center have identified 3 tumor-suppressor genes that reduce human lung cancer growth in mice. They are hoping that by injecting the genes into a patient's lung tumor, cancer cells will die or at least grow more slowly.

In addition to vaccination and gene therapy, taking a medication to reduce the risk of developing cancer in the first place is a relatively new approach to cancer management. A number of drugs are being tested to see if they can reduce the risk of lung cancer in people at high risk (mainly smokers and people who smoked for many years before quitting).

PULMONARY EMBOLISM

A pulmonary embolus is a blockage in 1 or more of the arteries in the lungs. In almost all cases, it occurs when a blood clot originating in a deep vein in the legs, arms, or pelvis breaks loose and travels to the lungs. Depending on its size, the blood clot, or embolism, obstructs a large or small pulmonary artery within the lungs and blocks the flow of blood through that vessel. Estimates suggest that more than 600,000 people in the United States suffer a pulmonary embolism each year, and about 10% of cases are fatal. Fortunately, steps can be taken to prevent pulmonary emboli.

Pulmonary embolism varies in its severity and effects. Most dangerous is an acute, massive blood clot that blocks a main pulmonary artery and/or 1 of its branches. Another dangerous situation is when a small blood clot blocks a peripheral pulmonary artery (one near the surface of the lung). Some people have multiple clots that block many medium-sized pulmonary arteries but produce no symptoms. The network of blood vessels in the lungs is large enough to tolerate considerable amounts of obstruction, but such extensive blockage can increase resistance to blood flow through the pulmonary arteries, eventually producing pulmonary hypertension (high blood pressure in the pulmonary arteries). Pulmonary hypertension places excessive stress on the heart's right ventricle, which pumps blood into the pulmonary arteries. This can lead to right heart failure.

Causes

The vast majority of pulmonary emboli are caused by blood clots from a deep vein in the leg, pelvis, or arm (deep vein thrombosis, or DVT). Each year, an estimated 5 million people in the United States suffer an episode of DVT. The condition is most common among women and older people.

A frequent cause of DVT is stagnation of blood flow, often seen in bedridden people who are immobile or healthy people who sit still for an extended period, such as on a long trip. Women taking oral contraceptives or hormone replacement therapy after menopause are at increased risk for DVT. People are at high risk for DVT after any major surgery, but especially after knee- or hip-replacement surgery.

A tendency for the blood to coagulate (change from a liquid to a solid state) can predispose a person to DVT. Having cancer also can cause the blood to coagulate excessively. In addition, injury to blood vessels by trauma, intravenous catheters or needles, or certain medications can cause blood clots.

Symptoms

Pulmonary emboli may produce sudden and severe shortness of breath, rapid breathing, and chest pain. Massive emboli, which often result in death within a few minutes, may also be accompanied by a

NEW RESEARCH

Genetic Factors Contribute to Lung Cancer Risk

First-degree relatives of people with lung cancer have a 2–3.5 times greater risk of developing lung cancer than the general population, according to a new study. The heightened risk associated with heredity extended well beyond the immediate family, the results indicate.

Researchers examined the contribution of genetic factors to the risk of developing lung cancer in the population of Iceland. The risk of developing lung cancer for parents of a lung cancer patient was 2.7 times greater than that of the general population; for siblings, the risk was 2 times that of the general population; and for children of lung cancer patients, 1.96 times the risk.

Risk increased among second-degree relatives, too: 1.34 for aunts and uncles, and 1.28 for nephews and nieces.

Even cousins, who are third-degree relatives, had 1.14 times the risk of the general population.

Genetic factors clearly play a major role in lung cancer risk. But it's noteworthy that tobacco was found to play a significant adverse role in lung cancer development, even among people genetically predisposed to it.

JOURNAL OF THE AMERICAN MEDICAL ASSOCIATION
Volume 292, page 2977
December 22/29, 2004

Palliative Care for Lung Cancer

When comfort is paramount

If lung cancer progresses and starts spreading to vital organs, it's time to make some difficult decisions. People with advanced lung cancer will need to talk with their doctor about whether they want to continue receiving aggressive treatment to control their cancer.

If a person's general health is good enough to withstand the side effects of more chemotherapy, he or she may decide to pursue further treatment. If, however, for reasons of health, finances and/or quality of life, the person decides not to receive chemotherapy any longer, then it's time to discuss palliative care. This is care that relieves suffering and improves quality of life so that a person can remain comfortable and continue to do some of the activities that make life pleasurable.

Pain Control

Pain is a major problem in people with advanced lung cancer, affecting an estimated 75% of patients. The causes of this pain include tumor growth and related nerve damage, toxic side effects of chemotherapy and radiation, and muscle aches when patients limit their physical activity.

Fortunately, in most patients with advanced lung cancer, effective pain management is possible. For mild to moderate pain, the first treatment of choice is a nonsteroidal anti-inflammatory drugs (NSAIDs) or acetaminophen, unless the doctor determines the patient should not be using these drugs. If pain persists or becomes worse, an opiate such as morphine is added—not substituted (using opiates and NSAIDs together often provide more potent pain relief than using either drug alone). Unfortunately, many doctors and patients are reluctant to use opiates because of concerns regarding addiction.

Other drugs that may be added include:

- Corticosteroids to lift mood, relieve inflammation, and reduce swelling of the brain or spinal cord
- Anti-seizure drugs to manage nerve pain
- Antidepressants to help manage nerve pain and elevate mood
- Tranquilizers to treat bone pain.

Management of Pain from Cancer that has Spread

When lung cancer has spread to the bone, external radiation therapy is typically recommended to control pain. Sometimes the steroid prednisone is given in combination with radiation for pain relief. Bisphosphonates (such as Zometa) are medications given alone or with radiation treatment to control bone pain. In patients whose health is fairly good, the doctor may consider surgery to stabilize the bone and minimize risk of fracture. Radiation and steroids may be given when lung cancer has spread to the brain.

Treatment of Breathing Problems

People with lung cancer may have shortness of breath or trouble breathing for many reasons. They may have COPD or another lung disease not related to the cancer. Other common reasons include the cancer itself, fluid in the lungs, airway obstruction, obesity, side effects of chemotherapy or radiation therapy, pneumonia, or not being able to move.

Medical therapies may include:

- Treating any co-existing lung diseases that may be causing breathing problems
- Giving the patient oxygen, bronchodilators, corticosteroids,

feeling of impending doom, profuse sweating, loss of consciousness, shock, and a bluish color in the lips and fingertips. Peripheral emboli, which also occur abruptly and without warning, are associated with chest pain and coughing up blood. People with multiple small emboli may have no symptoms for many months until they develop right heart failure, which can cause fatigue, swelling of the ankles, weight loss, and shortness of breath.

Deep vein thrombosis can cause pain and swelling in the affected body part, and the area may be tender and feel hot to the touch; however, because the condition usually occurs deep within the leg, about half the time there are no signs or symptoms. Often, DVT is discovered only when a physician looks for it in someone who is at high risk for the condition.

antibiotics or opiates

- Teaching breath control, activity pacing and relaxation techniques
- Giving opiates to control cough.

A person who continues to suffer from persistent pain despite everything the doctor tries to do should ask to be referred to a clinic that specializes in the management of pain. Pain control specialists are trained to find additional methods that may provide relief.

Other Problems to Report to the Doctor

People with advanced lung cancer also commonly experience fatigue, depression, anxiety, lack of appetite, and confusion. These problems should be reported to the doctor. The steps recommended to relieve fatigue in lung cancer patients are similar to those used to conserve energy in patients with COPD (see page 22). Depression and anxiety can be treated with a combination of medications and psychotherapy.

Where is Palliative Care Given?

Lung cancer patients who need palliative care may be cared for at home, in the hospital, or in an inpatient hospice. A patient who is cared for at home must have resources available, such as family members and home care attendants who have the physical and emotional strength to provide such care.

Patients and their families who are deciding between hospital and hospice care have many factors to consider. Be sure to weigh visiting hours and how much privacy is provided in the decision-making process.

Hospice Care

Typically, patients are eligible for a hospice program when they have about 6 months to live. The goal of a hospice is to help people live their last days with dignity and quality, surrounded by loved ones. Hospice care focuses on quality of life rather than length of life.

Hospice care is usually given in the home, but it can also be given in a hospital, nursing home, or private hospice center.

Cost of Palliative Care

Insurance policies vary widely in their treatment of palliative care. Check with your insurance company to find out which services are covered. Most health plans cover hospice care. Medicare has a special hospice benefit that covers the cost of care as well as medications.

The following are available to Medicare hospice recipients:

- Physician services for the medical direction of the patient's care
- Regular home visits by registered nurses and licensed practical nurses
- Home health aides and homemakers for services such as dressing and bathing
- Social work and counseling
- Medical equipment such as hospital beds
- Medical supplies such as bandages and catheters
- Drugs for symptom control and pain relief
- Volunteer support to assist patients and loved ones
- Physical therapy, speech therapy, occupational therapy, and dietary counseling.

For more information about the Medicare hospice benefit, visit www.hospicenet.org/html/medicare.html. For more information about hospice and palliative care, visit the website of the National Hospice and Palliative Care Organization at www.nhpco.org. ■

Diagnosis

Although a pulmonary embolus is suspected when symptoms occur in a person with typical signs of DVT, often there is not enough evidence to make a definitive diagnosis. Tests that may help the doctor diagnose DVT include an electrocardiogram—a recording of the electrical activity of the heart. Measurements of arterial blood gases (oxygen and carbon dioxide) may also aid in making a diagnosis.

Probably the most effective noninvasive test is a pulmonary isotope ventilation/perfusion (V/Q) scan. This test involves the intravenous injection of particles labeled with a radioactive substance. The particles become trapped in the small pulmonary blood vessels, and an external detector is used to locate the radioactivity. In healthy lungs, radioactivity is evenly distributed throughout the lungs. However, if the blood supply to a portion of the lung has been blocked by a blood clot, there will be no radioactivity in that area. The diagnosis of a pulmonary embolus is highly unlikely when a V/Q scan is normal.

Spiral CT scanning of the chest is increasingly being used to evaluate people with suspected pulmonary embolism. Studies suggest that it can accurately diagnose large and medium-sized pulmonary emboli, but not small ones.

The most definitive diagnostic test is an angiogram of the pulmonary arteries—an x-ray following the injection of a contrast material into the pulmonary artery. An angiogram is an invasive procedure and is performed only when the results of other tests are insufficient to guide therapy.

Prevention

The only effective way to prevent pulmonary emboli is to prevent the development of DVT and to recognize and treat DVT vigorously when it does occur. Steps to prevent DVT include taking frequent walks when on long trips, getting out of bed as soon as possible after any surgery, and using anticoagulants and other therapies (for example, pneumatic compression stockings) when possible if you are bedridden or have had a surgical procedure. People with a family history of DVT should take special precautions, as they may have inherited an abnormal tendency for their blood to clot. Moreover, individuals who have had DVT in the past are at increased risk for a recurrence.

Treatment

Supportive treatment for someone with a large pulmonary embolus includes pain relief and oxygen. "Clot-busting" drugs (thrombolytic agents) may dissolve the clot and restore blood flow through the blocked pulmonary artery. Surgical removal of the blood clot may be required if a person has a large life-threatening clot or if his or her condition deteriorates during medical treatment. Thrombolytic therapy and surgery are generally reserved for people with massive clots and shock. Most of the time, however, people with a pulmonary embolus are treated with anticoagulants—heparin and warfarin (Coumadin)—in both the short and long term. Intravenous heparin is started immediately and continued for at least 5 days, and oral warfarin is continued for 3–6 months (with close monitoring).

Unfortunately, anticoagulants are ineffective for preventing further emboli in some people and can be dangerous in people who are at high risk for bleeding in the head (people with a brain aneurysm, for example) or people with active gastrointestinal bleeding. In these instances, a sieve-like filtering device may be placed in the inferior vena cava (the vein that returns blood from the lower body to the heart) to prevent blood clots from entering the heart and lungs. Filters are also useful for people who have had recurrent bouts of pulmonary emboli. These devices become obstructed over time, but the flow of blood is not significantly affected because blood can be carried back to the heart through smaller blood vessels, called collateral vessels, which also develop over time around the obstruction. Continued use of anticoagulants is needed because clots can still reach the lungs through these new blood vessels.

INFECTIONS

The respiratory tract has a remarkable defense system to protect against the numerous potential hazards we breathe in each day, but sometimes bacteria, viruses, or other microorganisms overwhelm this defense system and cause a respiratory infection. There are many different types of respiratory infections, the most common of which include acute bronchitis, flu, and bacterial pneumonia.

The signs and symptoms of a lung infection can overlap with those of a noninfectious lung disease, making diagnosis difficult. In fact, people with noninfectious lung diseases are at increased risk for respiratory infections, either from the lung disease itself or its treatment (corticosteroids, for instance). Conversely, a respiratory infection may cause both scarring of the lungs and a decline in lung function, setting the stage for future and recurrent episodes of lung infection.

Acute Bronchitis

Acute bronchitis refers to inflammation of the bronchi. When these large airways are infected, they become inflamed and plugged with mucus.

Causes. Bronchitis usually is caused by a viral infection, typically a cold virus. It can also be triggered by exposure to chemical fumes, dust, smoke, or other air pollutants. Cigarette smokers and people with heart failure or obstructive lung disease (such as asthma or COPD) are at increased risk for acute bronchitis.

NEW RESEARCH

Nicotine Patches and Lozenges Can Help Even Heavy Smokers

Nicotine patches and lozenges are effective smoking cessation aides, even for heavy smokers, a new study shows.

Studies of nicotine replacement therapy (NRT) generally do not analyze or compare the effectiveness of NRT products relative to smoking rate or degree of nicotine dependence. This has left open the question of whether these products are effective for very-heavy smokers (at least 40 cigarettes a day) or highly-dependent smokers.

Researchers examined data from 2 randomized clinical trials of NRT. In the first study, 249 smokers received a nicotine patch and 253 received a placebo (dummy patch). In the second study, 450 smokers were given nicotine lozenges and 451 were given a placebo lozenge. Participants in both studies received intensive behavioral treatment.

The researchers found that the nicotine patch and lozenge significantly increased the 6-month rate of continuous non-smoking in both very-heavy smokers and highly-dependent smokers.

Given that very-heavy and highly-dependent smokers have the lowest chances of success when it comes to quitting, yet suffer the gravest consequences if they don't, these findings are particularly encouraging.

JOURNAL OF SUBSTANCE ABUSE TREATMENT
Volume 28, page 49
January 2005

Symptoms. The predominant symptom of acute bronchitis is a persistent cough that may produce gray, green, or yellowish phlegm. The cough may be preceded by a headache, fever, sore throat, or other symptoms typical of the common cold. Severe coughing bouts may produce chest pain. Other symptoms include breathing difficulties and wheezing. In healthy adults, the symptoms of bronchitis generally disappear on their own within a few days.

Diagnosis. A diagnosis is based on the signs and symptoms. A chest x-ray may be needed to rule out other lung disorders, but acute bronchitis itself does not produce any abnormalities that can be seen on an x-ray.

Prevention. The most important thing you can do to prevent acute bronchitis is to not smoke. You can reduce your chances of picking up a cold virus by washing your hands frequently after contact with people who may be infected, minimizing how much you touch your eyes and nose, and avoiding exposure to people with respiratory infections.

Treatment. Usually no treatment other than smoking cessation is necessary for acute bronchitis (see the feature on the next page). Sometimes dextromethorphan syrup and an albuterol inhaler are used, but antibiotics and antihistamines appear to have no effect when the acute episode is due to a viral infection. In people with chronic pulmonary disease, such as asthma, COPD, cystic fibrosis, or interstitial lung disease, a viral infection that destroys the protective layer of cells lining the trachea and bronchi may lead to a bacterial infection, which can worsen the underlying lung disease or lead to pneumonia. In these individuals, an attack of acute bronchitis would be treated with antibiotics.

Influenza

Influenza, or the flu, is an acute infection usually involving the upper respiratory tract. Outbreaks of influenza occur each winter and last for 2–3 months, leading to infection in 10–20% of the population. Influenza can worsen the symptoms of COPD and asthma. It can also make a person more prone to a bacterial infection that causes pneumonia, or the flu virus itself can cause pneumonia.

Causes. The cause of flu is a viral infection. Flu A virus is responsible for most of the outbreaks and causes more severe disease and more deaths than flu B or C.

Symptoms. Flu produces the well-recognized symptoms of the flu—headache, fever, and muscle aches, often accompanied by

Before You Take Antibiotics for Bronchitis, Consider This

Overuse can lead to antibiotic resistance

Many people who develop bronchitis go to their physician assuming they'll receive antibiotics to clear up the problem. But a recent study found that people with bronchitis or other uncomplicated lower respiratory tract infections who take antibiotics for their condition have little difference in relief of symptoms compared with patients who don't take antibiotics.

The study, published in the *Journal of the American Medical Association,* included 807 patients with bronchitis or a similar uncomplicated lower respiratory tract infection. It did not include patients with chronic lung disease or suspected pneumonia. Participants were randomly assigned to receive either immediate antibiotics, no antibiotics, or delayed antibiotics if symptoms had not gone away after 10 days.

Compared with immediate antibiotics, giving patients either no antibiotics or delayed antibiotics was associated with little difference in the duration or severity of symptoms. On average, patients were ill for 3 weeks in total; taking antibiotics reduced moderately bad symptoms an average of only 1 day. "It is difficult to justify widespread antibiotic prescribing for uncomplicated lower respiratory tract infection on this basis given the dangers of antibiotic resistance," the researchers concluded.

The researchers also found that the approaches of not offering antibiotics or using delayed antibiotics were both acceptable to most patients.

"I hope that this study makes physicians think more carefully about prescribing antibiotics to patients with bronchitis and other uncomplicated lower respiratory infections," says Peter B. Terry, M.D., author of this White Paper and Professor of Medicine, Division of Pulmonary and Critical Care Medicine, Johns Hopkins University School of Medicine.

Dr. Terry notes that a number of studies over the last several decades have clearly shown that about half of cases of acute bronchitis are caused by a virus. "Since antibiotics don't work against viruses, then in these patients, taking an antibiotic won't alter the natural course of their illness." But, Dr. Terry adds, some patients with bronchitis have bacteria growing in their airways and then become infected with a virus that encourages the bacteria to multiply, leading to pneumonia. "These patients will respond to antibiotics," Dr. Terry says. "The problem becomes how to know when a patient's bronchitis is viral or not. That's where a doctor's judgment comes in." Absence of a fever and clear or light yellow phlegm usually suggests the illness is viral, while fever, and dark yellow or green sputum that is thick and sticky is more suggestive of bacterial infection.

A doctor also needs to take into account the age and general health of the patient, according to Dr. Terry. "There are certain considerations a physician has to think about very carefully. If you're young and healthy and get acute bronchitis, you are likely to have a strong enough immune system to fight it off. But if you have severe chronic obstructive pulmonary disease [an infection that further narrows already damaged airways and compromises lung function], physicians tend to be more conservative with these patients. A doctor knows that a patient with borderline lung function is at risk of ending up in the hospital, possibly on a ventilator, so there is very little room for error. In these cases a doctor is more likely to prescribe antibiotics to be on the safe side." ■

chills, cough, sore throat, and weakness. Acute symptoms usually last for 2–5 days.

Diagnosis. A diagnosis of flu is made when a flu outbreak is present in the community and a person's complaints fit the pattern of symptoms.

Prevention. The Centers for Disease Control and Prevention (CDC) recommends annual flu shots for high-risk individuals to prevent flu or at least reduce its symptoms when it does occur. The high-risk group includes people aged 65 and older, those with lung diseases (such as COPD or asthma), and people with certain chronic illnesses.

A needle-free, nasal spray form of the flu vaccine, called FluMist, became available in late 2003, but this version is approved only for healthy people between the ages of 5 and 49. It contains weakened, live flu viruses instead of inactive viruses. These weakened strains usually do not cause illness because they have lost their disease-causing properties, but there is a small possibility that they can still reproduce and cause disease, especially in people with weakened immune systems. FluMist is therefore not recommended for people who are not healthy. In addition, studies with FluMist have not included enough patients over the age of 49 to determine whether this group responds differently than younger individuals. The safe and effective use of FluMist in people 50 years and older is not yet known.

The antiviral drugs amantadine (Symmetrel) and rimantadine (Flumadine) are effective in preventing flu during an outbreak in 70–100% of high-risk people who did not receive the flu vaccine. Another antiviral drug, oseltamivir (Tamiflu), was recently approved for prevention of flu in adults and adolescents. Too few studies have been done in older people or those with chronic illnesses to say whether it is effective in these groups, but it does not appear to be harmful.

Treatment. People with flu should get plenty of rest and drink lots of fluids. Over-the-counter products, such as decongestants, antihistamines, and pain relievers may relieve symptoms. Although antibiotics may be helpful when flu is complicated by a bacterial infection, these drugs have no impact on the flu virus itself.

Certain prescription medications can shorten the duration of flu if taken soon after symptoms appear. Amantadine and rimantadine can reduce symptoms by about half if administered within 48 hours of the appearance of symptoms. About 10% of people have central nervous system side effects, such as anxiety and jitters, when treated with amantadine. These problems are less common with rimantadine. Because of the side effects and the inconsistent effectiveness of these drugs, the recent availability of 2 other antiviral therapies, oseltamivir and zanamivir (Relenza), is an important development. Oseltamivir is an oral medication; zanamivir is inhaled. Use of these drugs early in the illness (within the first 2 days of the appearance of symptoms) has been associated with an improvement in symptoms and a milder infection.

Pneumonia

Pneumonia is an infection of the air sacs and surrounding lung tissue. It is the sixth leading cause of death overall and the primary cause of death from infectious disease in the U.S., claiming the lives of about 65,000 Americans each year. Most fatalities occur in people over the age of 65, who often have underlying disorders that increase their susceptibility to infection. Others at high risk for pneumonia include people with lung cancer or a suppressed immune system (for example, people with HIV or those who take immunosuppressive medications).

Based on x-ray results, the various types of pneumonia are often divided into those that affect a single lobe (lobar pneumonia) and those that occur as patches in several lobes (multi-lobar pneumonia). In addition, pneumonia may involve either 1 lung (unilateral) or both lungs (bilateral).

Causes. Hundreds of different microorganisms can infect the lungs. Viruses and bacteria are the most common infectious agents that cause acute pneumonia, but other organisms (such as *Mycoplasma pneumoniae, Mycobacterium tuberculosis,* fungi, and the parasite *Pneumocystis carinii*) can be responsible, especially if a person's immune defenses are compromised. Environmental exposure and the setting in which pneumonia occurs (for example, in the community, a nursing home, or a hospital) are major determinants of the type of pneumonia and the type of microorganism responsible for the disease.

The most common type of bacterial pneumonia is pneumococcal pneumonia, which is caused by the bacterium *Streptococcus pneumoniae.* Pneumococcal pneumonia can spread from person to person (by coughing, for example), especially when people live in close quarters, as is the case in nursing homes, military barracks, and prisons. Most people who develop pneumococcal pneumonia have some underlying disease (the bacterium *Streptococcus pneumoniae* is actually commonly present in the throats of healthy people). The underlying disease may be an acute infection like flu, but more often it is a chronic condition such as diabetes, alcoholism, cirrhosis, AIDS, a lung disease such as COPD, or a blood disorder like leukemia. Also at increased risk are cigarette smokers and individuals who are chronically malnourished or debilitated. Pneumococcal pneumonia is far more common in the elderly: The number of cases per 100,000 people ranges from 20 in young adults to 280 in people over the age of 75.

Half of all pneumonia cases are caused by viruses, not bacteria. Most often, viral pneumonia is a complication of flu, especially in older adults and those with other health problems. Like bacterial pneumonia, a virus that causes pneumonia can spread through close contact with an infected person.

NEW RESEARCH

Measuring Hormone Levels Can Cut Antibiotic Use for Pneumonia in Half

Measuring levels of the hormone procalcitonin in people with pneumonia can help doctors reduce the number of days a patient has to take antibiotics to get well, according to a new study. Procalcitonin test results can be obtained in just an hour.

Many cases of pneumonia are caused by bacteria; in these cases, procalcitonin is elevated and antibiotic treatment is required. But other cases of pnuemonia are viral and are therefore not helped by antibiotics. To avoid delaying treatment, however, doctors typically start all patients on antibiotics, which must be taken for 10–14 days.

The researchers studied more than 300 patients with pneumonia and gave half standard antibiotic treatment. The other half had their procalcitonin levels tested; 15% had very low procalcitonin levels and were presumed to have viral pneumonia and received no antibiotics. The remaining 85% had high levels and received antibiotics. The researchers measured their procalcitonin 4, 6, and 8 days later, and discontinued their antibiotics if their levels were low.

Patients with high procalcitonin who received antibiotics were able to stop after an average of 6 days. Their recovery and number of days hospitalized was similar to those who received a full course of antibiotics.

AMERICAN THORACIC SOCIETY INTERNATIONAL CONFERENCE
Abstract 325
May 2005

Most cases of viral pneumonia are mild and get better on their own. People at risk for more severe cases include the elderly, young children, and people with impaired immune systems (such as transplant recipients or people with HIV). People with viral pneumonia may also develop a bacterial infection, which can make their illness more serious.

Symptoms. In bacterial pneumonia, symptoms typically begin abruptly. They may include a cough that produces yellow phlegm, high fever, chills, sharp chest pain brought on by breathing or coughing, and shortness of breath. Young people usually have increased breathing and heart rates and appear acutely ill. Older adults, however, typically have fewer symptoms, experiencing lethargy and confusion but often no fever, and sometimes no lung-related symptoms.

The early symptoms of viral pneumonia may resemble those of infection with the flu virus: a dry cough; fever; headache; muscle pain; and weakness. Twelve to 36 hours later, however, people with viral pneumonia may experience increased breathlessness, worsening cough with mucus, high fever, and, possibly, blueness of the lips. People with very serious viral pneumonia may have extreme difficulty breathing.

Diagnosis. The initial diagnosis of all types of pneumonia is made from a person's medical history, physical examination, and chest x-ray, which may show a variety of abnormalities. The organism responsible for the pneumonia can be identified by examining a person's phlegm under a microscope. Ideally, a phlegm sample should be obtained before treatment, but treatment should not be delayed while waiting for the phlegm to be analyzed.

Other routine laboratory tests in people with suspected pneumonia include a blood cell count, measurement of electrolyte levels in the blood, urinalysis, liver function tests, and blood cultures. In bacterial pneumonia, the white blood cell count is typically high, though it can fall in severe cases. By contrast, in viral or mycoplasma pneumonia, the white cell count tends to be lower or normal.

Prevention. Although most types of bacterial pneumonia cannot be prevented, the pneumococcal vaccine is effective against 88% of the bacterial strains of Streptococcus pneumoniae, preventing 60–70% of pneumococcal pneumonia cases. Flu vaccine reduces the risk of viral pneumonia.

The CDC recommends vaccination against both pneumococcal pneumonia and flu for the following people: anyone aged 65 or older; people with chronic cardiovascular or lung disorders (but

Medicare Now Covers Counseling for Smoking Cessation for Many Seniors

The Centers for Medicare and Medicaid (CMS) recently added coverage for smoking and tobacco use cessation counseling for certain seniors. Now Medicare beneficiaries can receive coverage if they have an illness caused or complicated by tobacco use, including:

- heart disease
- cerebrovascular disease
- lung disease
- weak bones
- blood clots
- cataracts.

Medicare beneficiaries are also covered for smoking cessation counseling if they take any of the many medications whose effectiveness is complicated by tobacco use, including insulin and medicines for high blood pressure, blood clots, and depression.

Medicare covers counseling sessions only, not the cost of nicotine patches and gum or other products designed to help smokers quit. The policy covers 2 quitting attempts each year; each attempt has a maximum of 4 sessions. In other words, a maximum of 8 sessions in a 12-month period is covered.

The Centers for Disease Control and Prevention (CDC) estimates that about 9% of Americans aged 65 years and older smoke cigarettes, and that more than half of them report a desire to quit. According to the American Medical Association, studies have shown that seniors who try to quit smoking are 50% more likely to succeed than all other age groups, and seniors who do quit can reduce their risk of death from heart disease to that of nonsmokers within 2–3 years after quitting.

"Unfortunately, many people successfully quit smoking only after they develop symptoms of smoking-related diseases, such as a shortness of breath from COPD," says Peter B. Terry, M.D., author of this White Paper.

When counseling his patients to quit smoking, Dr. Terry uses a strategy that he and other physicians have developed over several decades. This strategy, outlined below, works best in conjunction with nicotine replacement products such as the patch or gum, and sometimes in combination with the drug buproprion (Wellbutrin). The key elements to quitting are:

- **Pick a quit date.** The smoker selects a date to cease smoking a few weeks in the future.
- **Determine smoking patterns.** "In the intervening weeks, we determine when the individual smokes, so that he or she can see the relationship between smoking and certain behaviors," Dr. Terry says.
- **Develop alternative strategies.** Once the patient identifies various patterns in their smoking habits, Dr. Terry works with them to develop alternative activities to do during the time they would normally smoke. "If the patient knows they usually smoke after breakfast while having coffee, he or she will develop an alternative ahead of the quit date, such as getting on the treadmill right after breakfast, or taking a half-hour walk."
- **Get rid of all smoking reminders.** The night before the quit date, the person gets rid of all smoking-related items in their home.
- **Reward each success.** Individuals develop a goal for themselves, such as going out to dinner with their spouse after they've been smoke-free for a certain period of time.

Quitting smoking is difficult, Dr. Terry acknowledges. "But I hope that Medicare coverage will encourage more people to do it—before they develop lung disease." ■

not those with asthma who are otherwise healthy); people with diabetes or chronic liver or kidney disease; and those with a suppressed immune system due to cancer chemotherapy or to conditions such as leukemia, multiple myeloma, or HIV.

Even people who have already had pneumococcal pneumonia should get the pneumococcal vaccine; a *Streptococcus pneumoniae* infection may confer immunity to one particular strain of the bacterium, but an infection with another strain is still possible. While the vaccine used to only be given once, a booster is now recommended every 5 years for people who were first vaccinated before age 65. The flu vaccine should be given every Fall, and it is safe to get at the same time as the pneumococcal vaccine.

Treatment. The treatment for pneumonia depends on the

cause. Because of practical difficulties in obtaining adequate phlegm samples and the delays in getting back the results, antibiotic treatment is often started immediately, based on the physician's suspicions of the most likely cause. Whether treatment requires hospitalization depends on the severity of the pneumonia, the individual's overall health status, and the availability of family members and other caregivers to take care of the person at home.

Antibiotics are the mainstay of treatment for bacterial pneumonia (as well as for some other types, such as mycoplasma pneumonia). The sooner treatment is started, the better. The antibiotic of choice depends on the type of bacteria responsible for the pneumonia. At one time, penicillin was highly effective against *Streptococcus pneumoniae*, but penicillin-resistant strains have become more common; newer antibiotics may be needed to treat highly-resistant strains. In addition, because mycoplasmas and other less common microorganisms may be the cause of the pneumonia (and the resulting symptoms may overlap with those of pneumonia caused by *Streptococcus pneumoniae*), combinations of antibiotics are generally used.

Antibiotics are not effective against viral pneumonia. Most people with viral pneumonia recover without treatment in 1–3 weeks. Humidified air, supplemental oxygen, and increased fluids may be advised. With treatment, symptoms typically improve rapidly. The speed of recovery usually depends on a person's previous health status. For hospitalized people with bacterial pneumonia, an early switch from intravenous to oral antibiotics (as symptoms improve) has been found to be safe and effective, enabling individuals to go home sooner. Improvements evident on chest x-rays typically lag behind symptom improvement, especially in older people with multi-lobar pneumonia, COPD, or alcoholism. ■

GLOSSARY

acute—Having a short and relatively severe course.

acute bronchitis—Inflammation of the bronchi.

alpha$_1$ antitrypsin—A naturally occurring substance in the body that protects against damage to the walls of the alveoli by blocking the action of enzymes that break down proteins. A deficiency in this substance is one cause of emphysema.

alveoli—Tiny air sacs in the lungs. The walls of the alveoli contain capillaries, which absorb inhaled oxygen into the bloodstream and release carbon dioxide from the bloodstream into the lungs to be exhaled.

amiodarone—Generic name for Cordarone, a drug used to treat an irregular heart rhythm.

apnea—Cessation of breathing.

arterial blood gases—A measurement of the oxygen, carbon dioxide, and acidity of blood taken from an artery.

asthma—A disease characterized by inflammation and narrowing of the bronchi, making breathing difficult.

beta$_2$ agonists—The most commonly used type of bronchodilator, medication that opens airways by relaxing bronchial smooth muscles.

blood gases—Oxygen and carbon dioxide in the blood.

blood pressure—Pressure of blood against the walls of an artery.

breath training—Techniques that help a person with COPD control his or her breathing rate, decrease the amount of energy required for breathing, and improve the position and function of the respiratory muscles.

bronchi—Large airways in the lungs that branch from the trachea.

bronchiectasis—Persistent widening of the airways as the result of a lung disorder such as a lung infection, tumor, or cystic fibrosis.

bronchioles—Small airways in the lungs that branch from the bronchi.

bronchiolitis obliterans—Obstructive inflammation of the bronchioles.

bronchoalveolar lavage—Putting saline in the lung, then removing as much as possible to examine for abnormal cells or for infectious organisms.

bronchodilators—Medications that open airways by relaxing bronchial smooth muscles.

bronchoscopy—Passage of a thin, hollow, flexible tube through the mouth and windpipe to allow viewing of the main bronchial passages.

cannula—A 2-pronged device that connects to the oxygen canister or concentrator and rests just inside the nostrils.

catheter—A thin, flexible tube.

chronic—Persisting over a long period.

chronic bronchitis—A recurrent problem defined by coughing up phlegm nearly every day for at least 3 months of the year (for example, every winter) for 2 or more consecutive years.

chronic obstructive pulmonary disease (COPD)—A group of lung diseases, mainly emphysema and chronic bronchitis, characterized by an obstruction of airflow during exhalation.

coagulate—To change from a liquid to a solid state.

continuous positive airway pressure (CPAP)—A technique that involves wearing a nasal mask that delivers a steady stream of air to maintain airway pressure and keep the back of the throat open in people with sleep apnea.

cor pulmonale—Heart disease due to resistance of blood flow through the lungs; it often leads to right heart failure.

corticosteroids—Medications that reduce inflammation, for example, in the airways.

Cushing's syndrome—A condition that produces complications such as osteoporosis, high blood pressure, and roundness of the face.

cystic fibrosis—An inherited disease in infants, children, and young adults that causes the body to produce an abnormally thick, sticky mucus that clogs the lungs and leads to life-threatening lung infections.,

deep vein thrombosis—A condition caused by formation of a blood clot in a deep vein of the body, usually in the leg, pelvis, or arm.

diaphragm—The large, dome-shaped muscle located at the base of the lungs, separating the chest cavity from the abdomen. The diaphragm plays an important role in breathing.

diffusion capacity—A measurement of how well gas passes across membranes in the lungs.

elastin—A protein that makes the lungs elastic.

emphysema—A disease in which damage to the alveoli causes the lungs to lose their elasticity. People with emphysema are unable to move adequate quantities of fresh air through their lungs.

epiglottis—A flap of cartilage in the back of the throat that prevents food from entering the trachea.

FEV$_1$ (forced expiratory volume in one second)—A pulmonary function test that measures the amount of

GLOSSARY—continued

air expelled from the lungs in the first second of a forced exhalation.

fibrosis—A process by which inflamed tissue becomes scarred. Scarring in the lungs is called pulmonary fibrosis.

FVC (forced vital capacity)—A lung function test that is a measure of the total volume of air exhaled.

gastroesophageal reflux (GERD)—A condition in which stomach acid flows back into the esophagus.

hypercalcemia—Excessive blood levels of calcium.

idiopathic pulmonary fibrosis—Progressive scarring of the lungs in which the cause is unknown.

interstitial lung disease—A group of lung disorders that affect the supporting matrix of the lungs.

interstitium—The supportive tissue between the air sacs of the lungs.

larynx—Voice box.

leukotrienes—Cell products that may narrow bronchi and stimulate the production of mucus.

lobe—A section of the lung; the right lung has 3 lobes, while the left lung has 2.

lung volume reduction surgery (LVRS)—A surgical procedure in which lung tissue affected by emphysema is removed.

lung volume tests—Tests to measure the amount of air in the lungs.

lymph nodes—Small round shaped clumps of immune defense cells that help prevent the spread of infection and protect the bloodstream from viral and bacterial invasion.

mediastinoscopy—A procedure in which the structures behind the breastbone in the chest cavity are examined.

mesothelioma—Cancer involving the pleura (the membranes that cover the lungs).

metered dose inhaler (MDI)—A device used to inhale medications that delivers a highly concentrated amount of drug directly to the airways.

mucus clearance device—A small handheld device shaped like a pipe. Blowing into it creates vibrations in the chest that loosen mucus and helps medication to penetrate the lungs more easily.

nebulizer—A device that vaporizes liquid medication into a fine mist that can be inhaled easily.

nodules—Small lumps of tissue.

obstructive lung disease—Lung disease in which the airways are narrowed.

oxygen concentrator—An electric device that extracts oxygen from room air.

oxygen flow rate—The number of liters of oxygen that comes out of the cannulae per minute.

palliative treatments—Care aimed at delaying the progression of disease, relieving pain, and limiting disease complications, rather than curing the disease.

passive smoking—Inhaling the smoke from cigarettes smoked by others.

peak flow meter—A handheld device that measures how rapidly air flows out of the lungs.

pharynx—The back part of the throat.

pleura—The membranes that cover the outside of the lungs and the inside wall of the chest cavity.

pleural effusion—Fluid within the pleural space.

pleurisy—An inflammation of the pleura.

pneumonia—An infection in the lungs.

pneumothorax—Leakage of air into the space around the lung.

polysomnography—Sleep studies that monitor brain waves.

primary lung cancer—Lung cancer that originates in the lung.

pulmonary artery—The blood vessel that delivers oxygen-poor blood from the right ventricle of the heart to the lungs.

pulmonary embolism—A condition that occurs when a blood clot travels from a vein in the leg, pelvis, or arm and lodges in the pulmonary artery.

pulmonary fibrosis—Chronic inflammation and progressive scarring of the walls of the alveoli (the air sacs of the lungs). When the cause is unknown, it is called idiopathic pulmonary fibrosis.

pulmonary function tests—A group of procedures used to evaluate the status of the lungs and to confirm the presence of certain lung disorders.

pulmonary hypertension—Abnormally high blood pressure in the arteries of the lungs.

pulmonary isotope ventilation/perfusion (V/Q) scan—A test used to help diagnose a pulmonary embolism, which involves the intravenous injection of particles labeled with a radioactive substance and the inhalation of radioactive particles.

pulmonary rehabilitation—A comprehensive preventive healthcare program provided by a team of health professionals to help people cope physically, psychologically, and socially with COPD.

pulmonary sarcoidosis—An inflammatory disease in which granulomas, small areas of inflamed cells, appear in the lungs and adjacent lymph nodes.

pulmonologist—A lung specialist.

pulse oximetry—A non-invasive way to measure the level of oxygen in the blood using a sensor placed on the fingertip or earlobe that directs a beam of light through the tissue.

radon—A colorless, odorless gas formed naturally during the decay of uranium, found in rocks and soil.

resectable tumor—A tumor that can be removed in its entirety.

restrictive lung disease—Lung disease in which the ability of the lungs to expand is impaired.

right heart failure—Heart failure that mainly affects the right side of the heart, slowing the movement of blood through the heart and causing swelling of the liver and edema of the legs.

secondary lung cancer—Lung cancer that has spread to the lungs from another part of the body.

side-stream smoke—Smoke coming from the end of a burning cigarette.

sleep apnea—Temporary cessation of breathing during sleep, often leading to daytime sleepiness.

spacer—An attachment to a metered dose inhaler (MDI) that eliminates the need to release the medication and inhale simultaneously.

spiral computed tomography (spiral CT)—An imaging test that generates a series of cross-sectional images that may be used to create a three-dimensional image.

spirometer—An instrument used in a pulmonary function test; it records the total volume and rate of air being breathed out. This test helps to diagnose or assess a lung disorder or to monitor its treatment.

spirometry—Measurement of the volume of air forcefully exhaled by the lungs as a function of time.

staging—A system for determining how much cancer a patient has and how far it has spread.

systemic—Affecting the body as a whole.

total lung capacity—The amount of air in the lungs after maximal inspiration.

trachea—Windpipe.

uvula—The tag-like structure that hangs down from the back of the throat.

uvulopalatopharyngoplasty—A surgical procedure that increases the size of the upper airway by removing the uvula and part of the soft palate.

vena cava—The vein that returns blood from the upper and lower body to the heart.

ventilation—Movement of air (gases) in and out of the lungs.

ventricle—Lower chamber of the heart. The heart has a right and left ventricle.

x-ray—A procedure that uses invisible electromagnetic energy to produce images of bones, organs, and internal tissues.

HEALTH INFORMATION ORGANIZATIONS AND SUPPORT GROUPS

American Academy of Allergy, Asthma & Immunology
611 East Wells St.
Milwaukee, WI 53202
☎ 800-822-2762
414-272-6071
www.aaaai.org
Offers public education on allergies and asthma through children's books, tips brochures, videos, newsletters, and a Web site. Offers referrals for allergists and immunologists. Supports asthma and allergy research through grants to medical training programs.

American Association for Respiratory Care
9425 N. MacArthur Blvd., Ste. 100
Irving, TX 7503-4706
☎ 972-243-2272
www.aarc.org
Society of respiratory health professionals. Web site supplies respiratory health tips, quizzes, and links to other organizations.

American Lung Association
61 Broadway, 6th Fl.
New York, NY 10006
☎ 212-315-8700
www.lungusa.org
Oldest voluntary health organization in the United States. Funds and conducts research on all lung disorders, with a special emphasis on asthma. Institutes school and workplace educational programs; provides information on air quality and tobacco dangers.

American Thoracic Society
61 Broadway
New York, NY 10006-2747
☎ 212-315-8600
www.thoracic.org
International organization that funds research and education programs to improve patient care. Offers referrals to support groups and information on respiratory disorders. Provides educational materials and classes.

COPD-Support, Inc.
PMB 127
24123 Peachland Blvd., C-4
Port Charlotte, FL 33954
www.copd-support.com
On-line group offering e-mail lists, chat rooms, forums, and a newsletter for people involved with COPD. Dedicated to providing patients and caregivers with support, education, and a way to share ideas and solutions for dealing with this disorder.

The Canadian Lung Association
3 Raymond St., Ste. 300
Ottawa, ON K1R 1A3
Canada
☎ 613-569-6411
www.lung.ca
Canadian national not-for-profit health association funds medical research, provides health education and programs with a focus on lung diseases (such as asthma and COPD), tobacco, and clean air. Ten provincial Lung Associations offer programs for the one in five Canadians living with lung disease.

The National Emphysema Foundation
15 Belden Ave.
Norwalk, CT 06850
☎ 203-849-9000
www.emphysemafoundation.org
Nonprofit organization that supplies information on emphysema and other lung diseases. Web site provides articles and tips on quitting smoking. Affiliated with the Norwalk Hospital in Connecticut.

National Heart, Lung, and Blood Institute
P.O. Box 30105
Bethesda, MD 20824-0105
☎ 800-575-WELL/301-592-8573
www.nhlbi.nih.gov
Lead component of the National Institutes of Health for lung disease research; provides written information on noncancerous lung disorders (e.g., asthma, COPD, and cystic fibrosis).

National Lung Health Education Program (NLHEP)
9425 N. MacArthur Blvd., Ste. 100
Irving, TX 7503-4706
☎ 972-910-8555
www.nlhep.org
The mission of the NLHEP is to promote the early diagnosis of COPD and related disorders through the widespread use of spirometry. "Test Your Lungs, Know Your Numbers" is the motto of the NLHEP.

LEADING HOSPITALS FOR LUNG DISORDERS

U.S. News & World Report and the National Opinion Research Center, a social-science research group at the University of Chicago, recently conducted their 16th annual nationwide survey of 3,400 board-certified physicians in 17 medical specialties. The doctors nominated the hospitals that they considered to be the best from among 6,007 U.S. medical centers. This is the current list of the best hospitals for lung disorders, as determined by a combination of factors: doctors' recommendations from 2003, 2004, and 2005; federal death rates; and factual data regarding quality indicators, such as the ratio of registered nurses to patients and use of advanced technology. However, because the results reflect the doctors' opinions to some extent, they are partly subjective. Any institution listed is considered a leading center, and the rankings do not imply that other hospitals cannot or do not deliver excellent care.

1. **National Jewish Medical and Research Center**
   Denver, CO
   ☎ 800-222-LUNG (5864)
   www.njc.org
2. **Mayo Clinic**
   Rochester, MN
   ☎ 507-284-2511
   www.mayoclinic.org
3. **Johns Hopkins Hospital**
   Baltimore, MD
   ☎ 410-955-5000
   www.hopkinsmedicine.org
4. **Barnes-Jewish Hospital**
   St. Louis, MO
   ☎ 314-747-3000
   www.barnesjewish.org
5. **Massachusetts General Hospital**
   Boston, MA
   ☎ 617-726-2000
   www.mgh.harvard.edu
6. **University of Colorado Hospital**
   Denver, CO
   ☎ 303-372-0000
   www.uchsc.edu/patients
7. **University of California, San Diego, Medical Center**
   San Diego, CA
   ☎ 800-926-UCSD (8273)
   www.health.ucsd.edu
8. **University of California, San Francisco, Medical Center**
   San Francisco, CA
   ☎ 888-689-UCSF/415-476-1000
   www.ucsfhealth.org
9. **Duke University Medical Center**
   Durham, NC
   ☎ 800-ASK-DUKE/ 919-684-8111
   www.dukehealth.org
10. **Cleveland Clinic**
    Cleveland, OH
    ☎ 800-223-2273/216-444-2200
    www.clevelandclinic.org

JOHNS HOPKINS
MEDICINE

THE JOHNS HOPKINS WHITE PAPERS

Selected Medical Journal Article

AS-NEEDED STEROID THERAPY FOR MILD PERSISTENT ASTHMA

Although treatment guidelines for people with mild persistent asthma recommend daily "controller" therapy, prescription patterns suggest that most people with mild asthma only use their controller therapies intermittently. In *The New England Journal of Medicine* article we've selected to reprint this year, Homer A. Boushey, M.D. and his colleagues propose that people with mild asthma may be using their treatment intermittently because they feel fine most of the time and therefore don't perceive the need for daily therapy. The researchers decided to analyze whether using corticosteroid therapy on an as-needed basis (rather than a daily basis) could be an acceptable approach to treatment for people with mild persistent asthma.

The researchers enrolled 225 adults and divided them into 3 groups: 1 group received placebo medication and was told to start inhaled or oral corticosteroid therapy only when symptoms arose (the intermittent group); another group took a leukotriene-receptor antagonist (zafirlukast) daily; a third group took an inhaled corticosteroid (budesonide) daily.

After 1 year of treatment, the researchers looked at the 3 groups' morning peak flow (a sign of lung function), as well as frequency of asthma flare-ups, the degree of asthma control, the number of symptom-free days, and the quality of life. The data showed no clinically significant difference among the 3 treatment groups with respect to morning peak flow. Although patients reported 26 more days free from symptoms of asthma per year when treated with daily budesonide compared with other treatments, the frequency of asthma flare-ups did not differ significantly among the groups.

These findings suggest that an as-needed approach to the treatment of mild persistent asthma—i.e., symptom-driven intermittent treatment with inhaled or oral corticosteroids—may be a practical option. This strategy is not only less expensive, but it could decrease the long-term adverse effects of steroid therapy. Of course it's only a feasible strategy if we can be more sure it doesn't exacerbate mild asthma, and the researchers therefore call for a large-scale trial of this treatment approach.

The NEW ENGLAND JOURNAL of MEDICINE

ESTABLISHED IN 1812 APRIL 14, 2005 VOL. 352 NO. 15

Daily versus As-Needed Corticosteroids for Mild Persistent Asthma

Homer A. Boushey, M.D., Christine A. Sorkness, Pharm.D., Tonya S. King, Ph.D., Sean D. Sullivan, Ph.D., John V. Fahy, M.D., Stephen C. Lazarus, M.D., Vernon M. Chinchilli, Ph.D., Timothy J. Craig, D.O., Emily A. Dimango, M.D., Aaron Deykin, M.D., Joanne K. Fagan, Ph.D., James E. Fish, M.D., Jean G. Ford, M.D., Monica Kraft, M.D., Robert F. Lemanske, Jr., M.D., Frank T. Leone, M.D., Richard J. Martin, M.D., Elizabeth A. Mauger, Ph.D., Gene R. Pesola, M.D., M.P.H., Stephen P. Peters, M.D., Ph.D., Nancy J. Rollings, M.Ed., Stanley J. Szefler, M.D., Michael E. Wechsler, M.D., and Elliot Israel, M.D., for the National Heart, Lung, and Blood Institute's Asthma Clinical Research Network

ABSTRACT

BACKGROUND

Although guidelines recommend daily therapy for patients with mild persistent asthma, prescription patterns suggest that most such patients use these so-called controller therapies intermittently. In patients with mild persistent asthma, we evaluated the efficacy of intermittent short-course corticosteroid treatment guided by a symptom-based action plan alone or in addition to daily treatment with either inhaled budesonide or oral zafirlukast over a one-year period.

METHODS

In a double-blind trial, 225 adults underwent randomization. The primary outcome was morning peak expiratory flow (PEF). Other outcomes included the forced expiratory volume in one second (FEV_1) before and after bronchodilator treatment, the frequency of exacerbations, the degree of asthma control, the number of symptom-free days, and the quality of life.

RESULTS

The three treatments produced similar increases in morning PEF (7.1 to 8.3 percent; approximately 32 liters per minute; P=0.90) and similar rates of asthma exacerbations (P=0.24), even though the intermittent-treatment group took budesonide, on average, for only 0.5 week of the year. As compared with intermittent therapy or daily zafirlukast therapy, daily budesonide therapy produced greater improvements in pre-bronchodilator FEV_1 (P=0.005), bronchial reactivity (P<0.001), the percentage of eosinophils in sputum (P=0.007), exhaled nitric oxide levels (P=0.006), scores for asthma control (P<0.001), and the number of symptom-free days (P=0.03), but not in post-bronchodilator FEV_1 (P=0.29) or in the quality of life (P=0.18). Daily zafirlukast therapy did not differ significantly from intermittent treatment in any outcome measured.

CONCLUSIONS

It may be possible to treat mild persistent asthma with short, intermittent courses of inhaled or oral corticosteroids taken when symptoms worsen. Further studies are required to determine whether this novel approach to treatment should be recommended.

From the University of California at San Francisco, San Francisco (H.A.B., J.V.F., S.C.L.); University of Wisconsin, Madison (C.A.S., R.F.L.); Pennsylvania State University College of Medicine, Hershey (T.S.K., V.M.C., T.J.C., E.A.M., N.J.R.); University of Washington, Seattle (S.D.S.); Harlem Lung Center and Columbia University, New York (E.A.D., J.K.F., J.G.F., G.R.P.); Brigham and Women's Hospital and Harvard Medical School, Boston (A.D., M.E.W., E.I.); Thomas Jefferson University, Philadelphia (J.E.F., F.T.L., S.P.P.); and the National Jewish Medical and Research Center, Denver (M.K., R.J.M., S.J.S.).

N Engl J Med 2005;352:1519-28.

TREATMENT GUIDELINES RECOMMEND daily antiinflammatory therapy to control mild persistent asthma.[1,2] This recommendation for so-called controller therapy was prompted by studies reporting that such treatment improves physiological measures of airway obstruction (peak expiratory flow [PEF] and forced expiratory volume in one second [FEV_1]), the severity of symptoms, the frequency of exacerbations, and the quality of life[3-5] and was reinforced by reports that inhaled corticosteroid treatment may prevent progressive loss of pulmonary function.[6-8] However, analysis of pharmacy records suggests that most patients infrequently renew their prescriptions for controller medications (inhaled corticosteroids and leukotriene-receptor antagonists).[9]

We reasoned that patients with mild asthma may be using their treatment intermittently because they do not perceive the need for daily therapy. To analyze whether this strategy could be an acceptable approach to treatment in patients with mild persistent asthma, we modified a symptom-based action plan to guide the use of inhaled or oral corticosteroids when signs or symptoms of asthma worsened.[10] In a three-way study — the Improving Asthma Control (IMPACT) Trial — we compared the level of asthma control obtained with the use of this intermittent-treatment approach with that obtained with use of the intermittent-treatment plan plus daily treatment with a controller medication, either an inhaled corticosteroid (budesonide) or a leukotriene-receptor antagonist (zafirlukast). Morning PEF, a widely used and robust indicator of airflow obstruction, was the primary outcome indicator. Secondary outcomes included the frequency of asthma exacerbations, the number of days lost from work or school, the number of symptom-free days, asthma-related quality of life, and a panel of physiological and biologic measures of asthma activity.

METHODS

PATIENTS

Patients were recruited between February 2000 and May 2002 at six centers with the use of methods and equipment described previously.[11,12] The protocol was approved by the institutional review board of each center, and written informed consent was obtained from each participant. Inclusion criteria were physician-diagnosed asthma, an age of 18 to 65 years, and an FEV_1, measured more than four hours after the most recent use of a bronchodilator, that was at least 70 percent of the predicted value. All patients had an increase in the FEV_1 of at least 12 percent and at least 200 ml after the inhalation of albuterol or a fall in FEV_1 of at least 20 percent after inhaling a concentration of methacholine of less than 16 mg per milliliter (PC_{20}; lower concentrations indicate greater reactivity).

Exclusion criteria included cigarette smoking, respiratory tract infection or corticosteroid use in the previous six weeks, and hospitalization or two or more visits to the emergency department for asthma in the previous year. Patients qualifying at a screening visit were instructed in the use of an electronic peak flowmeter (AirWatch, ENACT Health Management Systems) and were given a diary to record morning and evening PEF, asthma symptoms, nocturnal awakenings related to asthma, and as-needed albuterol use. They were instructed to take one puff from a placebo-dispensing dry-powder inhaler (Turbuhaler, AstraZeneca), which was identical in appearance to the device used to dispense inhaled budesonide, and one placebo tablet (identical in appearance to zafirlukast) twice a day.

We enrolled patients only if their diary records and findings during visits in the next four weeks met the criteria for mild persistent asthma (self-treatment with a beta-agonist more than two days per week, nighttime awakenings related to asthma more than two days per month, or variability in the PEF of 20 to 30 percent). Apart from accepting a baseline FEV_1 as low as 70 percent of the predicted value, we excluded patients if they met any criteria for persistent moderate asthma (i.e., daily self-treatment with a beta-agonist, nighttime awakenings once a week, or more than 30 percent variability in PEF).[1] Enrollment also required at least 70 percent adherence to diary keeping, Turbuhaler use (by counting the number of doses remaining in the inhaler), and tablet use (established by pill counts and by electronic drug-exposure monitoring [eDEM, Aardex] of the time and date of each opening of the pill bottle).[13] PEF measurements were made and diaries were kept for four weeks during the run-in period, at the midpoint of the study, and at the end of the study.

PROTOCOL

On entry, all patients received 10 minutes of instruction in a symptom-based asthma treatment plan (details of the plan are provided in the Supplementary Appendix, available with the full text of this article at www.nejm.org). The plan called for patients to take open-label budesonide (800 μg twice daily) for 10 days or prednisone (0.5 mg per kilogram of body weight per day) for 5 days if their asthma symptoms worsened.[10] The patients' understanding of this plan was not formally evaluated, but they did receive a written summary of the plan, and the plan was reviewed briefly at each study visit.

After completing the run-in period, the patients were assigned to one of three parallel treatment groups: twice-daily oral placebo and inhalation of 200 μg of budesonide, twice-daily oral zafirlukast (20 mg) and inhalation of placebo, or twice-daily oral and inhaled placebo (intermittent treatment) (Fig. 1) (see the Supplementary Appendix for details of the procedures at visits). Treatment assignment was stratified according to center, and the use of an adaptive randomization scheme ensured balance with respect to PC_{20}, age, and racial or ethnic group.

Budesonide, zafirlukast, and matched placebos in identical delivery systems (pills or Turbuhaler) were donated by AstraZeneca. Representatives of the company reviewed and commented on the protocol but made no other contribution to its design, conduct, interpretation, or presentation.

The run-in and treatment phases both ended with a 10-to-14-day period of intense combined therapy, consisting of 0.5 mg of prednisone per kilogram per day, 800 μg of budesonide twice daily, and 20 mg of zafirlukast twice daily, plus treatment as needed with albuterol (540 to 720 μg), to eliminate any easily reversed causes of airflow obstruction affecting PEF or FEV_1.

At study visits, FEV_1 was measured, adherence to treatment was assessed, the degree of asthma control was assessed by means of a seven-item questionnaire (in which a score of 0 indicated no symptoms and a score of 6 severe symptoms),[14] medication-related side effects were assessed, and symptom-related impairment or discomfort was evaluated by means of the Asthma Symptom Utility

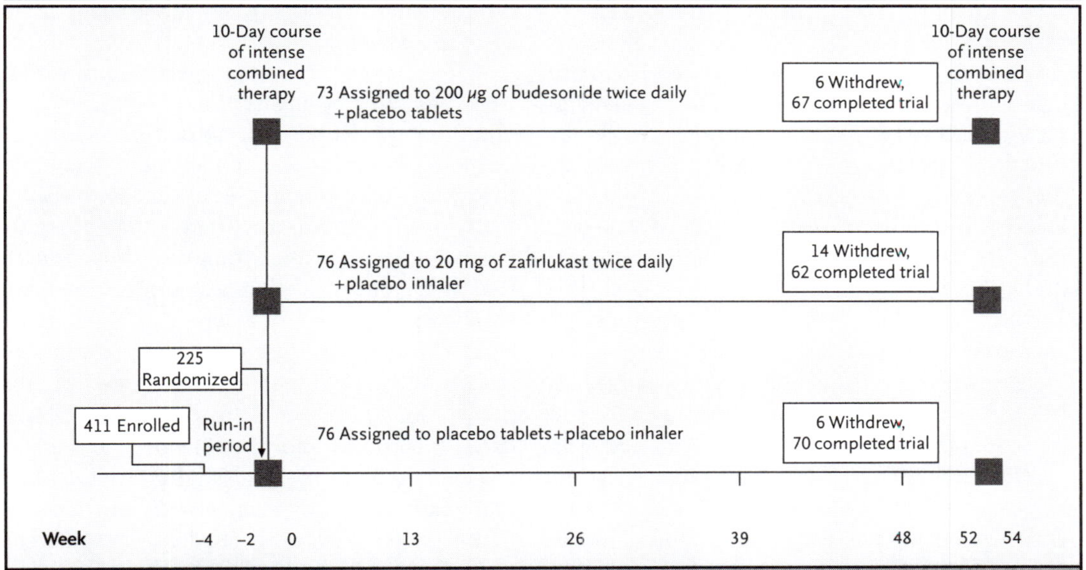

Figure 1. **Enrollment and Outcome.**

Reasons for exclusion during the run-in period were the need for inhaled budesonide therapy in 34 patients, excessive symptoms in 30, too few symptoms in 30, withdrawal of consent by 31, loss to follow-up of 19, failure to meet adherence criteria in 17, use of excluded medications by 6, presence of an excluded medical condition in 6, and other causes in 3. The run-in and treatment phases both ended with a 10-to-14-day period of intense combined therapy, consisting of 0.5 mg of prednisone per kilogram per day, 800 μg of budesonide twice daily, and 20 mg of zafirlukast twice daily, plus treatment with albuterol (540 to 720 μg), to eliminate any easily reversed causes of airflow obstruction affecting PEF or FEV_1.

Index.[15] The Asthma Symptom Utility Index is derived from a 10-item questionnaire completed by the patient. Scores range from 0 to 1, with higher scores indicating fewer symptoms. At visits during the periods in which diaries were maintained (four weeks during the run-in period and at the midpoint and end of the treatment periods, and during the two weeks of the two periods of intense combined treatment), peak flow was obtained from the diary records. Questionnaires about the number of symptom-free days, adverse events, and health care use were administered at all study visits and by means of telephone calls between visits. When these questionnaires identified patients who had had worsening of asthma symptoms, they were asked whether they had used the symptom-based action plan and this information was recorded.

The asthma-related quality of life was assessed by means of a questionnaire at enrollment and at the end of treatment[16]; patients rate the degree of impairment caused by asthma during the preceding 14 days and respond to each of the 32 items using a 7-point scale on which a score of 1 indicates maximal impairment and a score of 7 no impairment. Changes in the score of 0.5, 1.0, and 1.5 correspond to small, moderate, and large differences, respectively. The questionnaire can be used to provide an overall score and scores in four areas: limitation of activities, asthma symptoms, emotional functioning, and symptoms arising from environmental exposures. Exhaled nitric oxide, the PC_{20}, and the percentage of eosinophils in sputum were measured at enrollment and at the end of treatment (Fig. 1).

OUTCOME VARIABLES

The primary outcome variable was the change from baseline in two-week average morning PEF. Other objective outcome variables were the changes from baseline in the FEV_1 before bronchodilator use, the FEV_1 after treatment with 540 to 720 μg of albuterol, and the morning PEF during the period of intense combined therapy and FEV_1 after the period of intense combined therapy. We also measured the frequency of asthma exacerbations warranting the initiation of prednisone therapy according to the symptom-based action plan (whether initiated or not). Patients were instructed to notify their study center about these events, but we also identified such events by asking specific questions at study visits and during telephone contacts. Other patient-reported outcomes were responses to standard questionnaires on asthma control, asthma-related quality of life, symptom-free days, symptom-related impairment or discomfort, days missed from work or school, and adverse events (see above).

STATISTICAL ANALYSIS

The trial was designed to show the superiority of any one treatment over either of the other two. The primary outcomes were evaluated as the average percent change from the end of the run-in period to the end of treatment and were initially compared by means of analysis of variance. Pairwise comparisons between groups were evaluated if the P value for the overall test was less than 0.048 (by a two-sided test, adjusted for an interim analysis at the 0.005 level). These comparisons were then adjusted for baseline characteristics by including in an analysis-of-covariance model effects such as center, interaction between center and treatment, age, baseline PC_{20}, baseline FEV_1, duration of asthma, and other important baseline covariates listed in Table 1 (the list of covariates analyzed for each outcome is provided in the Supplementary Appendix). Repeated-measures analysis of covariance was also used on outcomes measured repeatedly throughout the study to evaluate correlated data.

The times to the first exacerbation of asthma were compared by means of Kaplan–Meier curves and the log-rank test. A repeated-measures proportional-hazards approach was used to compare groups, allowing for multiple exacerbations per patient.[17,18] The patient-reported outcomes regarding asthma control and symptoms throughout the trial were evaluated with repeated-measures analysis of covariance.

The primary end point compared among the groups was the change in morning PEF from randomization to the end of the trial. Using the standard deviation for morning PEF of 36.6 liters per minute noted in a previous study,[11] we calculated that a sample of 216 patients would provide a statistical power of 90 percent to detect the difference widely considered to be of clinical significance, 25 liters per minute, at a significance level of 4.8 percent, allowing a dropout rate of 15 percent. For the secondary end point — change in morning PEF from the first to the second period of intense combined therapy — we used the variability observed in the corticosteroid run-in period of a previous trial.[12] We calculated that if 199 patients completed the study, the study would have a statistical power of 80 percent to detect a difference of 21 liters per minute in this morning PEF during the period of intense combined therapy between any two treatment groups. We further calculated that this sample would provide 80 percent power to detect a change of 13 liters per minute in morning PEF within groups.

RESULTS

Of 411 patients who were enrolled after screening, 225 underwent randomization and 199 completed the study (Fig. 1). The treatment groups were well matched (Table 1). Twenty-six patients withdrew after randomization, 6 each from the budesonide and intermittent-treatment groups and 14 from the zafirlukast group (P=0.10). Reasons for withdrawal included loss to follow-up (in six patients), pregnancy (four patients), personal constraints (four patients), side effects possibly related to study medications (two patients), dissatisfaction with asthma control (one patient), and miscellaneous reasons (nine patients).

Adherence to study medication regimens, estimated from counting unused doses in the Turbuhaler and from pill counts and eDEM records, exceeded 90 percent and was similar among the groups. The use of open-label budesonide was no greater in the intermittent-treatment group than in the groups taking daily budesonide or zafirlukast (Fig. 2). Inhaled budesonide was taken for only 55 percent of the episodes of mild-to-moderate worsening of symptoms as defined by the asthma action plan (Supplementary Appendix). The average per-patient use of a daily controller medication over the year of the study was 47.8 weeks for the budesonide and zafirlukast groups (92 percent adherence × 52 weeks) and 0.48 week for the intermittent-treatment group.

The primary outcome, the change in morning PEF from the final two weeks of the run-in period to the final two weeks of the year of treatment, did not differ significantly among the groups, increasing about 7.8 percent (32 liters per minute) in all groups (P=0.90) (Table 2). The increases in average morning PEF from the first to the second period of intense combined therapy were also similar among the groups (3.5 to 5.7 percent, P=0.61) (Table 2), even after adjustment for center, age, minority status, and PC_{20}.

The pre-bronchodilator FEV_1 increased more in the budesonide group than in the other two groups (P=0.005) (Table 2), but the changes in

Table 1. Baseline Characteristics of the Patients.*

Characteristic	Daily Budesonide (N=73)	Daily Zafirlukast (N=76)	Intermittent Therapy (N=76)
Male sex — no. (%)	25 (34)	29 (38)	33 (43)
Minority — no.† (%) ‡	13 (18)	26 (34)	22 (29)
Black race — no.† (%)	9 (12)	11 (14)	13 (17)
Age — yr	33.2±9.5	33.6±11.1	32.0±10.5
Duration of asthma — yr	17.1±11.0	20.9±13.1	19.5±11.8
Data missing — no. of patients	2	2	5
Height — cm	170.0±10.4	170.3±8.9	170.2±9.6
Weight — kg	74.3±15.3	77.1±16.6	74.6±15.4
Body-mass index	25.7±4.4	26.5±5.0	25.7±4.6
Pre-bronchodilator FEV_1			
Liters	3.2±0.8	3.2±0.8	3.2±0.7
% Predicted	90.5±12.6	88.2±14.4	87.8±12.7
Morning PEF, 2-wk average — liters/min	467±117	468±111	462±106
PC_{20} — mg/ml§	1.08±1.25	1.33±1.43	1.17±1.22
Data missing — no. of patients	2	3	1
Exhaled nitric oxide — parts per billion			
Median	16.8	16.8	16.4
Interquartile range	11.7–25.1	10.5–24.9	10.3–23.5
Data missing — no. of patients	4	3	3
Sputum eosinophils — %			
Median	0.6	0.5	0.4
Interquartile range	0.2–2.0	0.0–1.3	0.0–1.3
Data missing — no. of patients	32	35	35
Asthma Quality of Life score¶	5.8±0.7	5.8±0.6	5.9±0.6
Asthma-control score‖	1.1±0.6	1.1±0.5	1.1±0.5
No. of symptom-free days in past 14 days	5.9±4.4	5.5±4.2	6.1±4.3
Asthma Symptom Utility Index score**	0.8±0.1	0.8±0.1	0.8±0.1

* Plus–minus values are means ±SD. To convert values for weight to pounds, multiply by 2.2. Body-mass index is the weight in kilograms divided by the square of the height in meters.
Minority status and black race were self-reported.
‡ P=0.07 by the chi-square test.
§ Geometric means and coefficients of variation are given.
¶ Scores can range from 1 (totally limited) to 7 (not at all limited).
‖ Scores can range from 0 (no symptoms) to 6 (severe symptoms).
** Scores can range from 0 to 1, with higher scores indicating fewer symptoms.

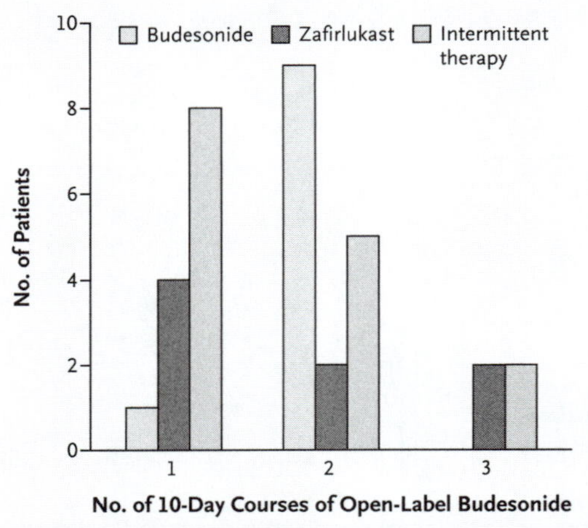

Figure 2. Number of 10-Day Courses of Open-Label Budesonide Initiated by Patients in Each Group, as Guided by the Symptom-Based Action Plan.

post-bronchodilator FEV_1 did not differ significantly among the groups (P=0.29) (Table 2). The average changes in post-bronchodilator FEV_1 in the budesonide and intermittent-treatment groups were −1.7 percent and −1.0 percent, respectively, resulting in an average difference between groups of −0.7 percentage point. The 95 percent confidence interval for this difference was −2.1 percent (i.e., greater decrease in the budesonide group) to 0.7 percent (greater decrease in the intermittent-treatment group).

The change in post-bronchodilator FEV_1 in the 46 patients with an FEV_1 at entry that was 70 to 79 percent of the predicted value was not significantly different from that in the 144 patients with an FEV_1 at entry that was at least 80 percent of the predicted value (P=0.59) (data not shown). The FEV_1 measured after the period of intense combined therapy declined similarly in all groups. Patients treated with budesonide had greater improvements in the percentage of eosinophils in sputum, exhaled nitric oxide values, and PC_{20} values than did the patients in either of the other two groups (Table 2). As compared with intermittent treatment, treatment with zafirlukast produced no significantly greater improvement in any outcome.

Thirty exacerbations of symptoms warranting treatment with prednisone occurred in 25 (11.1 percent) patients, an overall rate of 0.13 per patient-year. The proportion of patients who had one or more exacerbations did not differ significantly among the groups (one exacerbation in eight patients in the budesonide group and three in two patients in this group; one exacerbation in six patients in the zafirlukast group; and one exacerbation in seven patients in the intermittent-treatment group and three in one patient in this group).

Kaplan–Meier curves showed no significant differences among the groups, whether they were plotted as the time to a first event (P=0.39 by the log-rank test) (Fig. 3) or allowed multiple events per patient (P=0.24). The 12-month Kaplan–Meier exacerbation rates for the budesonide and intermittent-treatment groups were 16.1 percent and 11.3 percent, respectively, resulting in an average difference (i.e., positive sign indicates more exacerbations in the budesonide group) of +4.8 percentage points. The 95 percent confidence interval for this difference was −7 percent (lower in the budesonide group) to 16 percent (higher in the budesonide group). Patients initiated prednisone treatment for only 36.7 percent of the episodes (5 of 14 episodes in the budesonide group, 2 of 6 in the zafirlukast group, and 4 of 10 in the intermittent-treatment group). Five exacerbations required a visit to the emergency department (three in the budesonide group and one each in the other two groups). None warranted hospitalization. Altogether, patients missed 13 days from work or school because of asthma (7 days in the budesonide group, 2 days in the zafirlukast group, and 4 days in the intermittent-treatment group; P=0.18).

Of the patient-reported outcomes, the improvements in the asthma control score and in the number of symptom-free days were significantly greater with budesonide treatment than with either zafirlukast or intermittent treatment, which did not differ significantly from each other (Table 2). The greater number of symptom-free days over a 2-week period with budesonide (9.9 days) than with zafirlukast (8.7 days) or intermittent treatment (8.8 days) translates to 26 additional symptom-free days per year (95 percent confidence interval, 1.8 to 48.5). This was not associated, however, with any difference in the changes in the scores for the asthma-related quality of life, which improved in all groups (Table 2).

Neither the overall frequency of adverse events nor the frequency of severe events (36 or 37 in each group) differed significantly among the groups; seven of the patients with severe events required hospitalization. In this blinded study, no hospital-

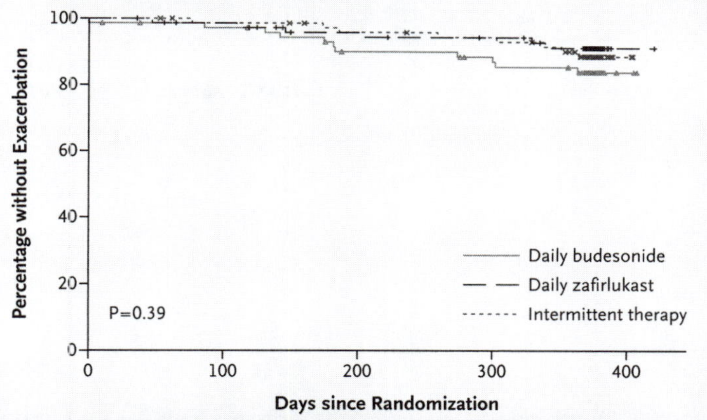

Figure 3. **Kaplan–Meier Estimates of the Time to a First Exacerbation of Asthma.**
There was no significant difference among the groups (P=0.39).

fer significantly among the groups. Although our study was not designed as a noninferiority trial and, thus, the findings must be considered preliminary, these data suggest that a novel approach to the treatment of persistent asthma — symptom-driven intermittent treatment with inhaled or oral corticosteroids — may be possible. Since the intermittent use of inhaled corticosteroids could decrease the adverse effects of these agents,[19] our data provide the impetus for a large-scale trial to test this novel approach to asthma treatment.

Epidemiologic studies have reported that the use of inhaled corticosteroids reduces asthma-related hospitalizations and deaths,[20,21] and some previous clinical studies of mild asthma have reported that inhaled corticosteroid therapy reduces the frequency of exacerbations and the rate of decline in the results of tests of airway caliber (PEF, FEV_1, or post-bronchodilator FEV_1),[3-5] so the suggestion that a large subgroup of patients with asthma may not require daily controller treatment will arouse concern.

However, the protective effect in the epidemiologic studies was most apparent by far in patients using frequent doses of an inhaled beta-agonist,[20] a pattern inconsistent with the criteria for mild persistent asthma. In our study of 411 patients who appeared on original screening to meet the criteria for mild persistent asthma, 64 were found to have asthma that was too severe and 30 asthma that was too mild to qualify. We believe that the lack of a difference among our treatment groups may reflect the low rate of exacerbations in patients who consistently meet the criteria for mild persistent asthma. This possibility is supported by our finding of a rate of exacerbations warranting prednisone treatment in our intermittent-treatment group (0.11 per patient-year) well below the rates reported in previous studies of mild asthma (0.21 to 0.77 per patient-year).[3-5]

This difference in asthma severity could also account for the difference from previous studies reporting that continuous corticosteroid therapy prevented a decline in airway function in patients with mild asthma.[3-5] We found no treatment-attributable difference in the change in post-bronchodilator FEV_1. Our study was shorter than the previous studies, but the preponderance of the differences between treatment groups in these studies occurred during the first year, and we noted no such effect. Our findings are consistent with those of the Childhood Asthma Management Program trial, a study of children with asthma, which showed no effect of five years of treatment with an inhaled corticosteroid on the change in post-bronchodilator FEV_1.[22] Furthermore, the robustness of our findings, as reflected by the confidence intervals for the differences in the decline in post-bronchodilator FEV_1 and in exacerbation rates, suggests that the treatment benefits that our study might have missed may be so small as not to justify the expense, potential adverse effects, and inconvenience of daily treatment with a controller therapy of all patients with mild persistent asthma.

We did find that budesonide (but not zafirlukast) improved markers of airway inflammation, such as bronchial reactivity, the percentage of eosinophils in sputum, and exhaled nitric oxide. It is noteworthy, however, that low-grade inflammation similar to that seen in our patients has been reported in patients with spontaneous, complete, sustained clinical remission of asthma,[23,24] who are not now considered candidates for daily controller treatment.

We found that daily treatment with budesonide (but not zafirlukast) was associated with a significant increase in the number of symptom-free days and a trend toward improvement in the scores for a weighted symptom utility index, but not in asthma-related quality of life. This lack of improvement in the quality of life may reflect the light burden of symptoms of mild asthma. In asthma of this severity, symptoms are occasional and are usually promptly relieved by treatment with an inhaled bronchodilator. Whether the increase in symptom-free days is worth the costs of treatment, both fiscal and

Table 2. Average Changes in Primary and Secondary Outcome Measures over a One-Year Period.*

Outcome	Daily Budesonide			Daily Zafirlukast			Intermittent Treatment			Overall P Value†
	No. of Patients	Value	Within-Group P Value	No. of Patients	Value	Within-Group P Value	No. of Patients	Value	Within-Group P Value	
Morning PEF (%)	66	8.3±1.9	<0.001	62	7.9±2.1	<0.001	70	7.1±2.0	<0.001	0.90
Morning PEF post-PICT (%)	66	5.7±1.7	0.002	62	5.6±1.8	0.002	69	3.5±1.7	0.05	0.61
FEV_1 (%)										
Pre-bronchodilator	67	4.0±1.2	0.001	62	−1.1±1.0	0.30	70	0.7±1.1	0.55	0.005
Post-bronchodilator	67	−1.7±0.5	0.002	61	−0.5±0.7	0.45	69	−1.0±0.5	0.04	0.29
Post-PICT	67	−1.5±0.7	0.03	62	−2.1±0.7	0.003	68	−0.6±0.6	0.34	0.27
Exhaled nitric oxide (%)	63		0.75	60		0.02	66		<0.001	0.006
Median		−14.4			12.4			26.6		
Interquartile range		−44.4 to 46.8		62	−24.6 to 82.8			−9.6 to 99.3	<0.001	
Sputum eosinophils (%)	34		0.03	26		0.71	35		0.03	0.007
Median		−0.3			0.0			0.2		
Interquartile range		−1.6 to 0.2			−0.9 to 0.3			−0.1 to 1.5		
PC_{20} (log_2)	63	1.8±0.2	<0.001	58	0.3±0.2	0.11	67	0.1±0.2	0.48	<0.001
Asthma Quality of Life score‡§	67	0.5±0.1	<0.001	64	0.3±0.1	<0.001	70	0.3±0.1	<0.001	0.18
Asthma control score‡¶	70	−0.4±0.1	<0.001	70	−0.2±0.04	<0.001	73	−0.3±0.05	<0.001	<0.001
No. of symptom-free days‡	70	4.0±0.4	<0.001	70	3.1±0.4	0.001	73	2.9±0.4	<0.001	0.03
Asthma Symptom Utility Index‡‖	70	0.06±0.01	<0.001	70	0.04±0.01	0.002	73	0.04±0.01	<0.001	0.06

* Unless otherwise stated, values reflect mean (±SE) changes from baseline to the end of the treatment period (before the period of intense combined therapy [PICT]) (see Fig. 1). In each analysis of covariance model evaluated to confirm the unadjusted results above, the covariates used in the stratified randomization scheme of the study were included (center, age, minority status, and PC_{20} value). All other baseline covariates listed in Table 1 were then considered to see whether they added any significant explanatory power to the model. In the resulting main-effects models, the interaction between center and treatment and all pairwise interaction terms of the predictors in each model were also considered. The results based on the inclusion of these factors in each model did not differ significantly from the conclusions of the unadjusted results reported above.

† P values refer to differences among the groups with the use of analysis of variance or repeated-measures analysis of covariance.

‡ Results are mean changes from baseline averaged over all visits; P values are from longitudinal analysis (repeated-measures analysis of covariance).

§ Scores can range from 1 (totally limited) to 7 (not at all limited).

¶ Scores can range from 0 (no symptoms) to 6 (severe symptoms).

‖ Scores can range from 0 to 1, with higher scores indicating fewer symptoms.

ization was deemed by the investigators as being related to the study, study medication, or asthma.

DISCUSSION

Our study of 225 patients with mild persistent asthma showed no clinically significant difference among the three treatment groups with respect to morning PEF. Although other objective measures of lung function and airway biology were improved and patients reported 26 more days free from symptoms of asthma per year when treated with budesonide on a daily basis than with the other treatments, the frequency of asthma exacerbations did not difwith respect to long-term side effects, may thus be an individual, subjective judgment best left to the patient and his or her health care provider.[19]

It is fair to ask whether the approach to treatment in our intermittent-treatment group could be practically applied outside of the artificial conditions of a clinical trial. We tried to mimic true clinical conditions by basing the action plan on symptoms, rather than on peak flow. All our patients were given an open-label budesonide inhaler, prednisone tablets, and 10 minutes of instruction in the symptom-based action plan. This instruction was reinforced by a written summary and by reminders of the plan at each visit and a telephone call (every six weeks). This attention to teaching an action plan might limit the generalizability of our findings. However, even under these conditions, patients took budesonide for only 55 percent of the episodes of mild-to-moderate worsening of symptoms and prednisone for only 37 percent of the episodes severe enough to warrant its use. We also found no significant difference in the rate of exacerbations warranting prednisone treatment in patients who should have but did not take budesonide (7 of 22) than in those who should have and did (15 of 21). Taken together, these observations suggest that close, formal adherence to the action plan may not have accounted for our findings.

In adults with long-standing, mild persistent asthma who were given medication and instructed to initiate corticosteroid therapy according to a symptom-based action plan, regularly scheduled controller treatment with either inhaled budesonide or oral zafirlukast had no significant effect on the rate of severe exacerbations, impairment in the quality of life, or the rate of loss of pulmonary function over a period of one year. These findings suggest that the novel approach of treating patients with mild persistent asthma with inhaled and oral corticosteroids as needed may be viable. Longer and larger studies will be needed before this approach to asthma treatment can be recommended.

Supported by grants (5 U10 HL051810, 5 U10 HL051823, 5 U10 HL051831, 5 U10 HL051834, 5 U10 HL051843, 5 U10 HL051845, and 5 U10 HL056443) from the National Institutes of Health.

Dr. Boushey reports having received consulting fees from GlaxoSmithKline and Aventis and lecture fees from GlaxoSmithKline and Genentech/Novartis; Dr. Sorkness, consulting fees from GlaxoSmithKline and lecture fees from GlaxoSmithKline, AstraZeneca, and Genentech/Novartis; Dr. Sullivan, consulting fees from AstraZeneca, Merck, Schering-Plough, and GlaxoSmithKline and lecture fees from AstraZeneca, Schering-Plough, and Pfizer; Dr. Fahy, consulting fees from Xoma Tularik, AstraZeneca, and Aventis; Dr. Lazarus, consulting fees from Merck, Schering, GlaxoSmithKline, and Critical Therapeutics and lecture fees from Boehringer-Ingelheim and Merck; Dr. Chinchilli, consulting fees from Wyeth and Procter & Gamble and lecture fees from Bristol-Myers Squibb and Aventis; Dr. Craig, consulting fees from Merck; Dr. Dimango, grant support from Genentech/Novartis; and Dr. Deykin, consulting fees from AstraZeneca, Genentech/Novartis, Intermune, and Roche; lecture fees from GlaxoSmithKline; and grant support from Merck. Dr. Fish is an employee of Genentech. Dr. Kraft reports having received consulting fees from Genentech/Novartis and AstraZeneca and lecture fees from Merck and Genentech/Novartis; Dr. Lemanske, consulting fees from Aventis and AstraZeneca and lecture fees from Aventis, AstraZeneca, Novartis, Merck, and GlaxoSmithKline; Dr. Martin, consulting fees and lecture fees from GlaxoSmithKline, Aventis, Merck, Ivax, and Genentech/Novartis and grant support from GlaxoSmithKline; Dr. Peters, consulting fees from AstraZeneca, Genentech/Novartis, Discovery, IDEC, Roche, RAND Corporation, and the Respiratory Disease Foundation; lecture fees from AstraZeneca, Genentech/Novartis, and Merck; and grant support from GlaxoSmithKline, Boehringer Ingelheim, Novartis, AstraZeneca, Pfizer, Altana, Centocor, and Abaris; Dr. Szefler, consulting fees from AstraZeneca, GlaxoSmithKline, Aventis, and Merck; lecture fees from GlaxoSmithKline and Genentech/Novartis; and grant support from Ross Pharmaceuticals and AstraZeneca; Dr. Wechsler, consulting fees from Merck and Genentech/Novartis; lecture fees from Merck, GlaxoSmithKline, and Genentech/Novartis, and grant support from Merck; and Dr. Israel, consulting fees from Merck, Schering-Plough, and Genentech/Novartis; lecture fees from Genentech and Merck; and grant support from GlaxoSmithKline, AstraZeneca, Genentech, and Merck.

We are indebted to Reuben Cherniack, M.D. (National Jewish Medical and Research Center, Denver), James P. Kiley, Ph.D. (National Heart, Lung, and Blood Institute, Bethesda, Md.), and Hector G. Ortega, M.D., Sc.D. (National Heart, Lung, and Blood Institute, Bethesda, Md.), for their valuable contributions to the design, conduct, and interpretation of this study.

REFERENCES

1. National Asthma Education and Prevention Program Expert Panel Report 2: guidelines for the diagnosis and management of asthma. Bethesda, Md.: National Institutes of Health, 1997. (NIH publication no. 97-4051.)
2. Global Initiative for Asthma. Global strategy for asthma management and prevention. Bethesda, Md.: National Institutes of Health, 2002. (NIH publication no. 02-3659.)
3. Haahtela T, Jarvinen M, Kava T, et al. Comparison of a $\beta 2$-agonist, terbutaline, with an inhaled corticosteroid, budesonide, in newly detected asthma. N Engl J Med 1991;325:388-92.
4. Pauwels RA, Pedersen S, Busse WW, et al. Early intervention with budesonide in mild persistent asthma: a randomised, double-blind trial. Lancet 2003;361:1071-6.
5. O'Byrne PM, Barnes PJ, Rodriguez-Roisin R, et al. Low dose inhaled budesonide and formoterol in mild persistent asthma: the OPTIMA randomized trial. Am J Respir Crit Care Med 2001;164:1392-7.
6. Haahtela T, Jarvinen M, Kava T, et al. Effects of reducing or discontinuing inhaled budesonide in patients with mild asthma. N Engl J Med 1994;331:700-5.
7. Selroos O, Pietinalho A, Lofroos A-B, Riska H. Effect of early vs late intervention with inhaled corticosteroids in asthma. Chest 1995;108:1228-34.
8. Agertoft L, Pedersen S. Effects of long-term treatment with an inhaled corticosteroid on growth and pulmonary function in asthmatic children. Respir Med 1994;88:373-81.
9. Stoloff SW, Stempel DA, Meyer J, Stanford RH, Carranza Rosenzweig JR. Improved

refill persistence with fluticasone propionate and salmeterol in a single inhaler compared with other controller therapies. J Allergy Clin Immunol 2004;113:245-51.
10. Côté J, Cartier A, Robichaud P, et al. Influence on asthma morbidity of asthma education programs based on self-management plans following treatment optimization. Am J Respir Crit Care Med 1997;155:1509-14.
11. Drazen JM, Israel E, Boushey HA, et al. Comparison of regularly scheduled with as-needed use of albuterol in mild asthma. N Engl J Med 1996;335:841-7.
12. Lazarus SC, Boushey HA, Fahy JV, et al. Long-acting beta2-agonist monotherapy vs continued therapy with inhaled corticosteroids in patients with persistent asthma: a randomized controlled trial. JAMA 2001; 285:2583-93.
13. Cramer JA, Mattson RH, Prevey ML, Scheyer RD, Ouellette VL. How often is medication taken as prescribed? A novel assessment technique. JAMA 1989;261:3273-7. [Erratum, JAMA 1989;262:1472.]
14. Juniper EF, O'Byrne PM, Guyatt GH, Ferrie PJ, King DR. Development and validation of a questionnaire to measure asthma control. Eur Respir J 1999;14:902-7.
15. Revicki DA, Leidy NK, Brennan-Diemer F, Sorensen S, Togias A. Integrating patient preferences into health outcomes assessment: the multiattribute Asthma Symptom Utility Index. Chest 1998;114:998-1007.
16. Juniper EF, Buist AS, Cox FM, Ferrie PJ, King DR. Validation of a standardized version of the Asthma Quality of Life Questionnaire. Chest 1999;115:1265-70.
17. Binder DA. Fitting Cox's proportional hazards models from survey data. Biometrika 1992;79:139-147.
18. SUDAAN software for the statistical analysis of correlated data, release 8.0.0. Research Triangle Park, N.C.: Research Triangle Institute, July 2001.
19. Allen DB, Bielory L, Derendorf H, Dluhy R, Colice GL, Szefler SJ. Inhaled corticosteroids: past lessons and future issues. J Allergy Clin Immunol 2003;112:Suppl 3:S1-S40.
20. Donahue JG, Weiss ST, Livingston JM, Goetsch MA, Greineder DK, Platt R. Inhaled steroids and the risk of hospitalization from asthma. JAMA 1997;277:887-91.
21. Suissa S, Ernst P, Benayoun S, Baltzan M, Cai B. Low-dose inhaled corticosteroids and the prevention of death from asthma. N Engl J Med 2000;343:332-6.
22. The Childhood Asthma Management Program Research Group. Long-term effects of budesonide or nedocromil in children with asthma. N Engl J Med 2000;343: 1054-63.
23. van den Toorn LM, Prins JB, Overbeek SE, Hoogsteden HC, de Jongste JC. Adolescents in clinical remission of atopic asthma have elevated exhaled nitric oxide levels and bronchial hyperresponsiveness. Am J Respir Crit Care Med 2000;162:953-7.
24. van den Toorn LM, Overbeek SE, de Jongste JC, Leman K, Hoogsteden HC, Prins JB. Airway inflammation is present during clinical remission of atopic asthma. Am J Respir Crit Care Med 2001;164:2107-13. [Erratum, Am J Respir Crit Care Med 2002;166:1143.]

CLINICAL TRIAL REGISTRATION

The *Journal* encourages investigators to register their clinical trials in a public trials registry. The members of the International Committee of Medical Journal Editors plan to consider clinical trials for publication only if they have been registered (see N Engl J Med 2004;351:1250-1). The National Library of Medicine's www.clinicaltrials.gov is a free registry, open to all investigators, that meets the committee's requirements.

NOTES

ISBN 1-933087-30-7
ISSN 1542-1961
Printed in the United States of America

JOHNS HOPKINS
MEDICINE

The Johns Hopkins White Papers are published yearly by Medletter Associates, LLC.

Visit our website for information on Johns Hopkins Health Publications, which include White Papers on specific disorders, home medical encyclopedias, consumer reference guides to drugs and medical tests, and our monthly newsletter *The Johns Hopkins Medical Letter: Health After 50*.
www.JohnsHopkinsHealthAlerts.com

The 2006 White Papers

Take Control of Your Medical Condition

JOHNS HOPKINS MEDICINE

66AWHP

Visit us online at www.JohnsHopkinsHealthAlerts.com/bookstore

YES, I've placed a check mark next to the White Paper(s) I'd like to receive for $19.95 each. Annual updates on each subject that I have chosen will be offered to me by announcement card. I need do nothing if I want the update to be sent to me automatically. If I do not want it, I will return the announcement card marked "cancel." I may cancel at any time. (Please add $2.95 for domestic, $4.95 for Canadian, and $15.00 for foreign orders to your total to cover shipping and handling.) (CT, FL, IL, MA and OH residents add sales tax.)

✔ Please put a check mark next to the White Paper(s) you wish to order.

001065	❑ Arthritis	$19.95	008060	❑ Prostate Disorders	$19.95
003061	❑ Coronary Heart Disease	$19.95	010066	❑ Digestive Disorders	$19.95
004069	❑ Depression and Anxiety	$19.95	011064	❑ Vision	$19.95
005066	❑ Diabetes	$19.95	012062	❑ Back Pain & Osteoporosis	$19.95
006064	❑ Hypertension and Stroke	$19.95	015065	❑ Memory	$19.95
007062	❑ Nutrition and Weight Control for Longevity	$19.95	019067	❑ Lung Disorders	$19.95
			020065	❑ Heart Attack Prevention	$19.95

METHOD OF PAYMENT: (U.S. funds only) ❑ VISA ❑ MasterCard ❑ Check Enclosed ❑ Bill Me

Name

Address

City State Zip

Credit Card # Exp. Date

Signature Date

Money Back Guarantee: If for any reason, you are not satisfied after receipt of your publications, return your purchase within 30 days for a full refund.

Detach and mail this card back to The Johns Hopkins White Papers, P.O. Box 420083, Palm Coast, FL 32142

The 2006 White Papers

Take Control of Your Medical Condition

JOHNS HOPKINS MEDICINE

66AWHP

Visit us online at www.JohnsHopkinsHealthAlerts.com/bookstore

YES, I've placed a check mark next to the White Paper(s) I'd like to receive for $19.95 each. Annual updates on each subject that I have chosen will be offered to me by announcement card. I need do nothing if I want the update to be sent to me automatically. If I do not want it, I will return the announcement card marked "cancel." I may cancel at any time. (Please add $2.95 for domestic, $4.95 for Canadian, and $15.00 for foreign orders to your total to cover shipping and handling.) (CT, FL, IL, MA and OH residents add sales tax.)

✔ Please put a check mark next to the White Paper(s) you wish to order.

001065 ❑ Arthritis $19.95 008060 ❑ Prostate Disorders $19.95
003061 ❑ Coronary Heart Disease $19.95 010066 ❑ Digestive Disorders $19.95
004069 ❑ Depression and Anxiety $19.95 011064 ❑ Vision $19.95
005066 ❑ Diabetes $19.95 012062 ❑ Back Pain & Osteoporosis $19.95
006064 ❑ Hypertension and Stroke $19.95 015065 ❑ Memory $19.95
007062 ❑ Nutrition and Weight Control for Longevity $19.95 019067 ❑ Lung Disorders $19.95
020065 ❑ Heart Attack Prevention $19.95

METHOD OF PAYMENT: (U.S. funds only) ❑ VISA ❑ MasterCard ❑ Check Enclosed ❑ Bill Me

Name

Address

City State Zip

Credit Card # Exp. Date

Signature Date

Money Back Guarantee: If for any reason, you are not satisfied after receipt of your publications, return your purchase within 30 days for a full refund.

Detach and mail this card back to The Johns Hopkins White Papers, P.O. Box 420083, Palm Coast, FL 32142

Johns Hopkins White Papers

Fold along this line and tape closed

NO POSTAGE
NECESSARY
IF MAILED
IN THE
UNITED STATES

BUSINESS REPLY MAIL

FIRST-CLASS MAIL PERMIT NO. 86 FLAGLER BEACH FL

POSTAGE WILL BE PAID BY ADDRESSEE

THE JOHNS HOPKINS WHITE PAPERS
PO BOX 420083
PALM COAST FL 32142-9264

Johns Hopkins White Papers

Fold along this line and tape closed

NO POSTAGE
NECESSARY
IF MAILED
IN THE
UNITED STATES

BUSINESS REPLY MAIL

FIRST-CLASS MAIL PERMIT NO. 86 FLAGLER BEACH FL

POSTAGE WILL BE PAID BY ADDRESSEE

THE JOHNS HOPKINS WHITE PAPERS
PO BOX 420083
PALM COAST FL 32142-9264

2006 WHITE PAPER TITLES

ARTHRITIS 2006 - Covers the three most common forms of arthritis–osteoarthritis, rheumatoid arthritis, and gout - as well as two other rheumatic diseases: fibromyalgia syndrome and bursitis.

CORONARY HEART DISEASE 2006 - Discusses four problems resulting from coronary heart disease: angina, heart attacks, heart failure and cardiac arrhythmias.

DEPRESSION and ANXIETY 2006 - Includes major depression, dysthymia, atypical depression, bipolar disorder, seasonal affective disorder, panic disorder, generalized anxiety disorder, obsessive–compulsive disorder, post-traumatic stress disorder, and phobic disorders.

DIABETES 2006 - Shows you how to manage your diabetes and avoid complications such as foot problems and vision changes. Reviews the latest tools for monitoring your blood glucose and the newest medications for controlling it.

DIGESTIVE DISORDERS 2006 - Covers gastroesophageal reflux disease, peptic ulcers, dysphagia, achalasia, Barrett's esophagus, esophageal spasm and stricture, gastritis, gallstones, diarrhea, celiac disease, constipation, Crohn's disease, ulcerative colitis, and colon cancer.

HYPERTENSION and STROKE 2006 - Explains how to treat your high blood pressure and prevent it from harming your health. Also covers the two forms of stroke: ischemic stroke and hemorrhagic stroke.

BACK PAIN and OSTEOPOROSIS 2006 - Addresses back pain due to sprains, strains, and spasms; degenerative changes of the spinal bones and disks; disk herniation; and spinal stenosis. Also covers osteoporosis, a common cause of fractures in the spine and hip.

LUNG DISORDERS 2006 - Includes information on emphysema and chronic bronchitis (together referred to as chronic obstructive pulmonary disease or COPD), asthma, pneumonia, lung cancer, and sleep apnea.

MEMORY 2006 - Tells you how to keep your memory sharp as you get older and how to recognize the symptoms of age-associated memory impairment, mild cognitive impairment, and illnesses such as Alzheimer's disease and vascular dementia.

NUTRITION and WEIGHT CONTROL for LONGEVITY 2006 - Gives you the information you need to eat a healthy diet and keep your weight under control. Also explains what to do when the pounds just don't seem to budge.

PROSTATE DISORDERS 2006 - Helps you decide among the various treatment options for prostate cancer, benign prostatic hyperplasia, and prostatitis.

VISION 2006 - Reviews the current knowledge on cataracts, glaucoma, age-related macular degeneration, and diabetic retinopathy. Also discusses ways to cope with low vision.

HEART ATTACK PREVENTION 2006 - Provides up-to-date strategies for preventing a first heart attack, including identifying possible risk factors, the latest screening tests, risk-reducing lifestyle measures, and medications for controlling cholesterol.